When AIDS Comes to Church

William E. Amos, Jr.

The Westminster Press
Philadelphia

Book design by Gene Harris

First edition

Published by The Westminster Press®
Philadelphia, Pennsylvania

PRINTED IN THE UNITED STATES OF AMERICA

9 8 7 6 5 4 3 2

Library of Congress Cataloging-in-Publication Data

Amos, William E., 1940–
    When AIDS comes to church / William E. Amos, Jr. — 1st ed.
        p.   cm.
    ISBN 0–664–25009–2 (pbk.)

    1. AIDS (Disease)—Patients—Pastoral counseling of. 2. AIDS (Disease)—Patients—Family relationships. 3. Church work with gays. 4. Church work with families. 5. First Baptist Church (Plantation, Broward County, Fla.) 6. Amos, William E., 1940–
7. AIDS (Disease)—Religious aspects—Christianity. I. Title.
BV4460.7A48 1988
259′.4—dc19   87–30875
                                                                             CIP

This book is lovingly dedicated to the people of the First Baptist Church of Plantation, Florida, whose understanding of the church as a community of faith has made all this possible.

Contents

Foreword

The visit with an elderly grandfather by his pastor, William Amos of Plantation, Florida, seemed routine—until the grandfather began talking about the death of a beloved grandson with AIDS. The visit was a harbinger of the need for this Christian pastor to become proficient in ministering to AIDS patients in the milieu of the congregation as a fellowship of believers.

This book is the odyssey of what happened to one pastor, his congregation, the AIDS patients, and the members of their families in the dire circumstances of this killer disease. The pages that follow are not the speculations of theorists quoting terrifying statistics. They document the human situations of specific individuals and families, a compassionate pastor in the trenches of pastoral ministry, and a down-to-earth congregation who genuinely became the body of Christ, caring for those afflicted with AIDS. William Amos researched the available knowledge on the subject of AIDS as he ministered to these persons, their loved ones, and the congregation. He conferred with experts in university medical centers and collaborated with other pastors who likewise are grappling with their pastoral responsibilities. He disciplined himself to write down what he was experiencing and learning as events happened around him and to him. The book you are now reading is the eyewitness account of those events and the distillation of William Amos's thoughts in the presence of God. He gives a remarkably candid account of his own feelings as he assimilated new experiences into his worldview, of his perceptions of himself as a minister, and of his conversations with God in prayer.

I have had the privilege of being one of many consultants for William Amos in his pilgrimage of caring for AIDS patients and in crafting this book. I have learned much I did not know about the nitty-gritty of the pastoral care of people with AIDS. I have learned that to dismiss these patients as uniformly homosexual can be a dangerous mistake. In New York City, for example, the *New York Times* estimates that 36 percent of people with AIDS are from the drug scene and are users of dirty hypodermic needles. Prostitution is a prevalent source of infection. Heterosexuals and the infants they produce are an increasing population. To consider AIDS solely as the plight of the homosexual obscures the prevalence of infection from dirty needles, heterosexual experiences, and yet-to-be discovered other sources of the scourge.

I also learned that from the angle of vision of Christ's compassion, the pastor and the congregation care for AIDS patients as they would any other dying patient with a lethal disease. They are not untouchables. "Touched by a human hand, and wakened by kindness, chords that were broken will vibrate once more" as Christian pastors and working churches convey the spirit of Christ. Poorly obscured by pious judgmentalism, the love of God breaks through and casts out fear.

This is a foretaste of the learning that awaits you as you read this remarkable pastoral story.

WAYNE E. OATES
Professor, School of Medicine,
University of Louisville, and
Senior Professor, The Southern
Baptist Theological Seminary

Preface

This book has been born out of day-to-day pastoral relationships in the First Baptist Church of Plantation, Florida. It is basically the story of how we responded as the people of God when AIDS came to our church. The families involved are all members of our congregation. The presence of AIDS in their lives provides the setting. Their presence in our church community provides the context. The response of the church is the story.

The names of the families who are dealing with AIDS have been changed at their request. Confidentiality remains an immensely important issue. Their names, as such, are of little consequence. Their presence—in the life of our church and in the pages of this book—is the important issue.

They have been and remain my teachers in this journey. In the midst of their struggle and suffering, they all remain one of God's really good gifts.

After two and a half years of responding through ministry in this suburban church to those dealing with AIDS, I am convinced that no other issue has the same potential as this disease to change the face of pastoral ministry. There will be families in the church who, because of their connection with the disease, will be viewed as untouchable. The issue of confidentiality will become more complex and demanding as the minister works with AIDS patients and their families. As AIDS spreads into the heterosexual community, more and more persons will be labeled with the scarlet letter of somehow improper sexual activity. Guilt, fear, and anger will surface in those whose lifestyles have involved activities that could result in AIDS. Pastoral issues will become paramount, in that the church will be faced with the reality that forgiveness of sin and consequences of sin are two different things when AIDS is involved. Premarital counseling will take on an entirely different flavor as the ethical and moral dimensions of one's past behavior are seen to affect one's present and future relationships.

If the spread of the disease even approximates the projections of the medical community, there is no question that the response of the church and its ministers will take on a different complexion than ever before. It is my hope and prayer that this book will help to raise the right questions, point in the right direction, and in some way more adequately prepare the church and its ministering family to provide the strongest and most redemptive response possible to those dealing with AIDS.

I especially want to acknowledge my deep gratitude to some individuals whose participation with me has made this book possible. I am especially indebted to my wife, Janette, for assuming the task of proofreading the manuscript and, more important, for serving so patiently and lovingly as my center of calm during this time. My son and daughter have quietly and consistently lent their support; my son's singular encouragement and belief in me kept me at the task of finishing this manuscript even when I was not sure I could. My secretary, Lynn Perry, has generously provided the ministry of concern in the typing of this manuscript.

Dr. Wayne Oates has given the marvelous gift of blessing and encouragement from the very beginning. His excitement and hope for this story to be told has been surpassed only by his careful, methodical guidance throughout the entire process. I have not only been greatly helped, I have been enriched beyond measure by his pastoral participation in this journey.

1

When AIDS
Came to Church

Like many other people when the first cases of AIDS were reported in this country in 1981, I was interested in this curious new disease. I read about it as information became available. I listened to reports as the issue became more a part of life in our society. But, also like so many others, I did not really claim much ownership of this problem.

Pastoring a church in South Florida meant living in one of the truly high-risk areas. The medical community was quick to identify two groups whose behavior put them at the highest risk of exposure to the disease: the gay and the drug communities. Fort Lauderdale, Miami, and the Florida Keys have become notorious for drug-related activities, and they also have a very large and well-established gay community. On more than one occasion in the early days of hearing and learning about AIDS, I felt that our community was surely going to have to deal with this strange disease. Yet at the same time, it was relatively easy to remain detached because of the nature of my own ministry.

The city of Plantation, Florida, is a delightful suburb of Fort Lauderdale. We are close enough to have access to the beautiful beaches and waterways for which Fort Lauderdale is famous. However, our location about seven miles inland means that we are far enough away to feel the smug security of a suburban community. Plantation is, without question, one of the better places to live in South Florida. In terms of its population, Plantation is also a very young city. The 1986 reports from the local Chamber of Commerce proudly describe the average age of the residents as about thirty-five. The average income is in the $32,000-to-$34,000 range. While many retired people live in South Florida, the city of Plantation has maintained the character of an upper-middle-class suburban community of young, upwardly mobile families.

In the midst of Plantation is the First Baptist Church, with a resident membership of about 600. Begun in 1960, it is only a few years younger than the city itself. The ministry of the church has always reflected the community in which it is located. As is true of the city of Plantation, there are not many older people. The population of the church consists mainly of young families, with an abundance of children and teenagers. The ministry and programs of the church reflect the needs both of this membership and of the community.

Any picture of this church as in the midst of the emerging AIDS dilemma seemed from the very beginning to be slightly out of focus. The church has always had a very open view toward struggling to bring the gospel to bear on all sorts of situations and needs. However, being open and being involved are two very different things. At best, we in the church expected to be involved from a distance. We would be open to concern about and awareness of the AIDS issue as a problem that was happening elsewhere. We certainly never expected AIDS to come to Plantation in general, and to the First Baptist Church in particular.

Dennis

My own introduction to AIDS came in a rather surprising way, on what seemed to be a normal pastoral visit. Late in 1984, one of our very special elderly members sustained the loss of an only grandson. I called to see if I might come by and visit with him. Dennis was then in his mid-eighties, very alert and as involved in church activities as his body would allow. After the death of his wife several years earlier, this gentleman farmer from the Deep South had reluctantly moved to South Florida. Being Baptist born and bred, he quickly found his way to our church and began quietly to endear himself to our church family.

We sat down together and started to talk. Dennis began with perhaps the point of greatest pain: His only grandson was dead, and with that death went his hopes for the continuation of the family name. Family was very important to Dennis, and the pain was obviously deep. The tears flowed as he talked about his loss.

Then, in his quiet gentle way, Dennis went on to say that he hoped his grandson had made his peace with God and had gotten his life straightened out in California. The boy had gone to San Francisco because he felt that the community there would be one into which he could fit more easily. Dennis explained that his grandson was gay and had died with AIDS. He was very careful to let me know of the depth of his love for his grandson, even though he did not understand or agree with his lifestyle. But he had read and heard enough about AIDS to know what a painful death his grandson had endured.

As we talked together, Dennis's concerns centered around two areas. The first was that he needed me as his pastor to know that he was hurting deeply as he experienced the loss of his grandson. The pain was especially poignant because, as Dennis reminded me, grandparents are not supposed to outlive their grandsons. Second, it was important for him to communicate to me his deep concern about his grandson's spiritual life. He repeated his hope and prayer that his grandson had "gotten things straight with God" before he died. Dennis had written him gently on more than one occasion about this concern.

In the midst of sharing this second concern, Dennis raised his head and looked me straight in the eye. "Pastor, I know what the Bible has to say about homosexuality. Do you think homosexual people can go to heaven?" There was a look of both pain and hope on this dear man's face.

Given the nature of the question and the nature of the

questioner, I knew there was no easy answer. For the next half hour, we talked about redemption and forgiveness and the need for hope. I assured him that homosexuality was not the unforgivable sin; alone, it would never keep anyone out of heaven. I believe that heaven will be filled with all kinds of forgiven sinners. The issue at hand was not the grading of various "sins" but how we choose to deal with the relationship of our lifestyles before God.

We prayed together and we wept together. Dennis was weeping for the loss of his grandson. I was weeping at the bravery of this man as he dealt with his pain.

Later that afternoon, I sat in my car in his driveway for a few minutes reflecting on the visit. God had allowed me the privilege of sharing a unique experience. This eighty-five-year-old man whose gay grandson died with AIDS was struggling boldly and honestly with what scripture said about this situation, and yet through it all he never once let the fact of his grandson's identity become a barrier between them. His love for him and his hope for him in eternity clearly overrode his feelings about the choice of lifestyle his grandson had made, however different it was from his own. Then I drove off, back into a world that would hardly acknowledge the presence of homosexuality or AIDS, much less talk about either subject with understanding and compassion.

Dennis now lives in a nursing home. At every visit, even though our communication is very different now, I thank God anew for this teacher, this friend, who helped prepare the way for all that was to come.

Tom and Ruth

My second encounter with AIDS came from within the congregation. Shortly before Christmas in 1984, one of our faithful members entered the hospital with a persistent respiratory illness of unknown origin. I was out of the city for the first few weeks of January but learned, upon my return, that Tom was still hospitalized. I immediately went to see him and was concerned to find him in isolation, looking really ill and quite thin.

He and his wife, Ruth, said that a group of infectious disease specialists had been called in to see what the problem was. Tom had developed a strange variety of pneumonia called *Pneumocystis carinii*. Could AIDS be the culprit? I wondered. Knowing Tom had once been involved with drugs heightened my fears, and a member of the church who was working in cancer research at the University of Miami Medical School agreed that all signs seemed to point in that direction.

Tom and Ruth and I are all very up-front people, and we talked openly about the possibilities. The doctors in Plantation also suspected AIDS and made a referral to the University of Miami clinic for confirmation of the diagnosis.

In struggling to acknowledge the reality of their situation, I reflected about the way this young couple had come into our lives at First Baptist Church. Early in 1981, Tom and Ruth began attending church services. Follow-up visits in their home led to the development of a really warm and significant relationship. Just before coming to our church, Tom had gotten involved in the Alcoholics Anonymous program and, as a part of working on his program of the "twelve steps," decided it was time to get his spiritual life in order. He and Ruth began looking for a church in which they could feel comfortable and be challenged to grow. After considerable discussion, prayer, and searching, Tom made his profession of faith and was baptized into the family of God and the fellowship of First Baptist Church on September 6, 1981. Ruth came with him, moving her membership from another church in the community.

Tom and Ruth quickly began to make a place for themselves in our church family. It was interesting to watch this happen, because they were different from the kind of folks who usually join our church. Neither of them were college graduates or part of the more typical upwardly mobile, management level of the Plantation community. Their excitement about their growing faith and relationships within the church community was refreshing, and our church welcomed them warmly.

Getting to know Tom and Ruth better was a fascinating experience from the very beginning. Knowing a bit of where they had come from, especially Tom, made their own excitement about their growing discipleship even more meaningful and contagious. Not only was Tom dealing with the problem of dependency on alcohol, he had also been extensively involved in the drug scene.

Tom grew up the rough way. He is what is often referred to as street-wise. A native of Pennsylvania, Tom decided at an early age that life was a giant buffet from which one could—indeed, should—sample at will. He tried it all: heroin, marijuana, cocaine, alcohol, crack, uppers, downers, a previous marriage to a prostitute, and a host of other things.

Arriving in Florida, Tom settled down to fun in the sun near the beautiful Atlantic Ocean. As a street-wise young man, he had learned to pay close attention to what was going on around him. Now, while running a charter boat during the winter season to Bimini, he met a man who offered him a berth on his seventy-five-foot schooner sailing through the Caribbean and to Central and South America. This fellow often left Tom in charge of the boat while he flew back to the States to attend to business matters. It was during these times that Tom met various "characters," as he called them. With them he visited many different places and experienced a host of things.

During his time in South America, Tom learned quite a bit about the drug trade. When he returned to the States, he was able quickly to find connections and put this new knowledge to work. His new business not only filled many hours but also satisfied much of his need for thrills, excitement, and danger, and he was making big money, as well.

After several of these adventures he met Ruth, and they began to date. Ruth did not know the details of Tom's life, but she became caught up in his excitement. They dated for about a year and a half. When Tom went away on "missions" from time to time, Ruth returned to her regular routine of living. Then they married and began to struggle with the process of settling down. They both acknowledge that for someone like Tom, this was not easy. Not long after they were married, Tom's drinking and drugs began to get out of control. Ruth, to use her words, "fell apart." By the grace of God, she found an organization called Al-Anon, which is that part of the Alcoholics Anonymous organization designed for the nondrinking spouse. Slowly, Ruth's life began to regain some semblance of sanity. Tom, in the meantime, played with AA, drifting in and out of the organization and its program.

Finally, after several roller-coaster years, Tom decided to get serious about AA's "twelve steps" program. Out of this experience, he and Ruth began to feel the need for a more personal expression of their faith in God. And so this fascinating and unusual couple came into our lives at First Baptist Church.

Not only did Tom and Ruth endear themselves personally to many people in the congregation, they began to assume leadership responsibility. Ruth started teaching in our Children's Division. Tom was asked to serve on the Building and Grounds Committee. This provided a perfect outlet for his really creative and ingenious abilities; there was not much that Tom could not do with his hands. It is important not to move too fast with people, especially those who are new in their discipleship, but for Tom and Ruth the timing really seemed right, and they were both most effective in what they did.

During this period of spiritual growth, the allure of his former life would sometimes overcome Tom, and he would slip back into old habits. Even during these up-and-down times, his commitment to his Lord, himself, and his church remained a constant force. In reality, Tom experienced what most of us experience; he felt more firmly rooted in his faith on some days than on others. The only difference was that Tom's dependency problems made the process much more acute and complicated than for most of us.

Knowing all this made the diagnosis of AIDS especially hard to accept. Since the virus can lie dormant for as long as nine years,[1] it is possible that Tom was exposed before he ever came into the church and the family of God. The exposure also could have happened during one of his times of struggle after his baptism. Either way, it seemed grossly unfair, because Tom and Ruth were both trying so hard to get things to work right.

From the very beginning, Tom and Ruth both handled the news of AIDS with a great deal of strength and faith. There was a quiet kind of acceptance on their part that when you choose to dance, the piper must be paid.

When he was discharged from the hospital in Plantation, Tom asked me to go with him to Miami for confirmation of the diagnosis; he wanted his pastor with him, for support and for understanding. There was never a question in my mind as to whether I would go or not. In addition to being there in a pastoral role for Tom and Ruth, I wanted some answers of my own. Perhaps some time with the doctors at the AIDS clinic would also be of help to me.

As I drove Tom and Ruth down to Miami, the atmosphere was heavy with what we all knew was ahead. The doctors in Plantation had been pretty definite in their diagnosis, but the needed confirmation could only be made through the clinic at the University of Miami. A friend and fellow church member, Kay, who worked in cancer research in the same general area of the AIDS clinic, had agreed to meet and guide us through this unfamiliar territory. As we walked toward the entrance to the clinic, I prayed that strength would be present for Tom and Ruth, to deal with the reality of what we knew was coming, and also thanked God for placing someone like Kay in their lives.

In fact, as Tom's disease progressed, this relationship with Kay and her husband deepened and grew truly significant. The two couples had met through church, long before Tom was diagnosed with AIDS. Kay and Tim's interest in boats was a natural connecting point for Tom and Ruth. Tom, the master sailor, taught them how to sail, helped them figure out what kind of boat to buy, and went with them on more than one sailing weekend. These two couples seemed an odd foursome. Here were Tom and Ruth, with their varied and colorful past full of experiences from the world of drugs and alcohol, developing a really special relationship with Tim and Kay, both of whom have earned doctorates. Tim has his degree in horticulture and works in research for the University of Florida, and Kay has hers in biochemistry and is in cancer research at the University of Miami Medical School. The hand of God was really apparent in this relationship.

Even in the midst of those circumstances that day, there was a genuine sense of "OK-ness" because of the way God's presence and love were revealed to us. God had given us the gift of one another. God had provided through the mystery of relationships a tightly knit network of people who would be able to support Tom and Ruth as they supported each other. Even when the difficulties in our lives are of our own making, God does not turn a judgmental and wrathful side toward us. The pieces were falling into place for the journey that was ahead. Those pieces all bore the distinct mark of the loving God.

As in most clinic settings, waiting is the first step. As we sat in the reception room, Kay explained in great detail how the results of the test would be stated and what they would mean. She helped us understand how the AIDS virus attacks the immune system. To have it all explained so clearly was reassuring. At least we had some sense of what the doctor would be talking about.

Finally, Tom went in. In a short while, the doctor called for Ruth and me. Dr. Dickinson, one of the leaders in the AIDS research at the university, dealt with both of them gently but clearly. He carefully outlined what was happening in Tom's body, and he talked specifically about what would happen when the body could no longer fight disease and infection. He described in detail the journey of AIDS patients in order to give Tom some idea of what was ahead. At the same time he was clear about what doctors did not know and what research was being done. This small word of hope, however dim it may have been, was grasped by Tom and Ruth in the way that drowning victims grab for a life ring.

Dr. Dickinson talked in detail about the changes in their lifestyle that would need to accompany the presence of AIDS. In nonalarming and practical terms, he outlined ways the disease could be communicated so they would know what adjustments needed to be made. The most obvious change would be in their sexual expressions to each other. Condoms would be required, and they would have to refrain from deep kissing so as not to get any exchange of body fluids. Since injected drugs were not now a part of their lives, precautions in this area were a moot point.

The normal patterns of living together—eating, sleeping, using the same bathroom—all were put into perspective. Dr. Dickinson dealt clearly and reassuringly with all the questions Tom and Ruth had brought. Tom had been especially afraid of communicating the disease to Ruth or to her daughter, who lived with them. Of course, this concern extended to others that he would be around.

It was so good to hear the doctor say that outside of the exchange of body fluids or blood, there was virtually no risk of infecting anyone else. Their anxiety dropped visibly. One area of concern, however, remained very high for them both, the fear that Ruth had already been infected. Obviously, in their normal sexual activities, Ruth had regularly been exposed through the exchange of body fluids. Not knowing exactly when Tom contracted the disease, the awareness of what might have happened during the time that had elapsed between his exposure and the discovery of the virus in his system was threatening to them both.

Tom got his courage up to ask Dr. Dickinson about Ruth and whether he had unknowingly infected her. Dr. Dickinson said it was certainly a possibility, and there was a test Ruth could take to confirm whether or not the AIDS virus was present in her system as well. Ruth said quietly that for the time being she was fine and was not interested in taking the test. Rather than run the risk of confirming at this point that she too might someday die with AIDS, she felt it was better not to know. Dr. Dickinson was sensitive to her feelings and simply indicated that whenever she wanted to have the test made, it could be done. The decision was up to her.

There was a question I wanted to have answered before we left the clinic that day. During my short involvement with the world of AIDS, I had already experienced what is called "AIDS hysteria" in the broader community: an overreaction on the part of people who were basically uninformed, frightened, or just plain prejudiced. There had been calls from parts of the South Florida area through the press for all AIDS victims to be openly identified, so that everyone who met them could avoid contact to prevent being infected. This demand sounded frighteningly similar to the tattooing of Jews by the Third Reich in World War II. On more than one occasion, persons with AIDS had been fired from their jobs because of the disease. Unfortunately, termination in these cases often had little to do with the actual physical effects of the disease and the person's ability to do the work. More often than not, in the early days, termination came as a result of intense pressure in the workplace from co-workers who were afraid to be around people with AIDS.

For this reason, I was deeply concerned about how to balance the reality of AIDS hysteria, and the confidentiality necessary to protect Tom's job, with this couple's need for emotional and spiritual support from the church community. I was optimistic about the overall response of our congregation, but there was a real risk of Tom and Ruth's being alienated from some of the very people whom they loved and from whom they needed continued support.

I voiced my concern to Dr. Dickinson. With all the authority and presence that medical people can muster, he told me in no uncertain terms that I had a responsibility openly to educate and inform the congregation about AIDS. The pulpit was a good forum for healthy education. He told me to let the congregation know I was involved with AIDS patients, and was not afraid, and they did not need to be afraid either. I had to risk being the recipient of AIDS hysteria myself. In this sense, I was being asked to put myself at risk in my pastoral relationships. Perhaps there would be people who would not come to church anymore when they found out about my ministering with AIDS patients. Perhaps there would be people who would not want me to visit in their homes and their hospital rooms. There was the distinct possibility that they would see me as an AIDS carrier.

I tried to digest all this and at the same time make the doctor understand the peculiar dilemma I faced. I was sure that if I could educate him to my special role he would have some magic insight about how I could be a really good pastor to Tom and Ruth and yet not risk anything personally with the congregation. Dr. Dickinson read my agenda like a book and cut through it with these words, now burned indelibly inside me. "Look, Reverend, the bottom line is this: I am not asking you to do anything that I am not doing—relating to AIDS patients in the context of my profession and then talking openly about it as a means of education. It's the only way to go, the only way. You need to know that I believe what I am telling you so completely that I am literally staking my life on it. Because if I am wrong, Reverend, I'm *dead* wrong."

Interestingly enough, I do not recall saying anything else. Indeed, it had all been said. We finished up the conference with some last-minute information for Tom in regard to his medication and then headed back home.

The ride back to Fort Lauderdale was quiet. Tom was processing the reality that he was going to die with AIDS. Ruth was dealing with that fact, plus her own need to decide when she would have the test to see if she had contracted the virus also. I was aware of their thoughts, but most of my energy was focused on the burden that Dr. Dickinson had laid on me: how to handle this in the congregation.

We talked about some of our concerns and agreed that at this point, since Tom was still well enough to work, confidentiality was a must. As a crane operator belonging to the local union, Tom could not disclose that he had AIDS; this would mean sure and swift dismissal. For Tom to become unemployed at this point would mean loss of insurance benefits as well as loss of income. The day would come soon enough when he would not be able to work.

This decision could be called "survival ethics." I believe in honesty and openness. However, the demands of this situation—Tom's need for income in order to survive and pay for medical treatment—meant that not fully disclosing all we knew was the only alternative. When Tom could no longer work, confidentiality would no longer be an issue. It would also be at that point, we all agreed, that he and Ruth would really need the help of the congregation.

In the weeks that followed, Tom and Ruth's life returned to normal as much as it could. Both of them went about their normal workdays, with the only differences being Tom's constant tiredness and his adjusting to a load of new and different medications. From a distance, they looked fairly normal. However, because of my closeness to them, I knew they were dealing with some really heavy concerns.

Tom expressed a strong need to talk his way through what he was feeling. I made a covenant with him that we would meet regularly to do this. Dealing with terminal illness and walking with people through the dying process is not new to any pastor who takes the calling seriously. The complexities and facets of AIDS began to fade into the background in the presence of the reality that here was a human being who was dying. What he was dying from and how he contracted the disease seemed less important at this point.

I was still faced with Dr. Dickinson's piercing words about dealing with the public side of AIDS, and after a great deal of prayerful thought and conversation, I went back to Tom and Ruth with a suggestion. I had concluded that I needed to preach from time to time on the subject of AIDS in the hope that my sermons could be used by God as a part of the healing process that families and churches and communities all needed to experience. I told

Tom and Ruth that I would always let them know in advance when I was going to mention AIDS in my sermon so they could decide ahead of time whether or not they wanted to be present. And I would make personal references to being involved with AIDS patients without specifically referring to Tom and Ruth.

In the weeks and months to come, my involvement in supporting Tom and Ruth took me to the AIDS center in Fort Lauderdale, where support groups met for AIDS patients. Tom and Ruth went to these meetings, and I went with them. I began to get involved in visiting AIDS patients in the hospital and in their homes. All this provided an excellent background for me to draw on in sermons. This way, I was able to provide what I felt was a real ministry and at the same time deal responsibly with the need for education in our church. Through it all, I was also able to maintain confidentiality for Tom and Ruth at this point in Tom's illness.

While continuing to work closely with Tom and Ruth, I somehow concluded that while AIDS had indeed come to our church, it came because of the unusual and somewhat unique circumstances of who Tom and Ruth were. Never did I consciously expect to continue to be confronted with other AIDS ministries.

Larry

The story for our church, however, was far from completed. Late in the summer of 1986, a church member came to me with the difficult and painful story of a family member who had AIDS. Then, less than six months later, in early 1987, yet another member stopped me on the sidewalk with the news that her family, too, had been touched with AIDS. Everything I had been hearing and reading about the spread of AIDS was becoming reality. In the short span of two years, four families had come forward in our congregation who had experienced or were experiencing what this disease is all about.

I met Larry through Emily, a relative of his who is a member of our church. Larry was twenty-six years old and gay. An only child, he had a large family of aunts, uncles, and cousins, most of whom were in the Bible Belt. Only his immediate family lived in South Florida. Naturally, they were very close.

When Emily came to speak with me about Larry's illness, her story did not come easily. She said she had wanted to talk to me for some time about Larry but was uneasy about discussing the matter with anyone. She simply was not sure how I would respond.

There was a good reason for her hesitation. When Larry began to identify with his feelings of homosexuality in his late teens, he approached his parents with the news. Church had always been a part of Larry's family experiences. Following Larry's disclosure about his sexual identity, they did what seemed natural to them and went to share their burden with their pastor. Unfortunately, what they experienced was not support but a quiet yet emphatic withdrawal of the church family. The young people who had been part of Larry's close circle of friends began to disappear into thin air. The message was clear. The pastor and the church were not at all comfortable in dealing with this family and their situation.

Naturally, Larry's family left that church community with deep feelings of hurt and anger. It was no wonder that Emily was sensitive about talking with her pastor. What finally convinced her to come and share with me was hearing me make several references to AIDS in general, and my role in particular, in sermons on Sunday mornings. Little did I know that God would use those instances of my speaking to the issue from the pulpit to pave the way for further ministry to those touched by AIDS.

Dr. Dickinson from the clinic in Miami had been right. Open discussion of this disease was indeed the only way to go. Had I not taken the risk of following his advice and counsel, Emily would probably never have come to me. It was reassuring to know that risk taking sometimes provides

opportunities for ministry that might never happen otherwise.

As I listened to Emily describe this part of the family's
story, it was apparent that the focus of her concern was
Larry. Her love for him was paramount. She, along with his
parents, deliberately chose not to let Larry's identity rob
her of an ongoing relationship with him. Within the immediate family, they were quite open about Larry's homosexuality. Their maturity in working through the pain that goes
with that kind of situation was apparent. It enabled them to
create a strong presence of love and support for him, and
this now was proving to be truly life-giving for Larry during
his illness.

Emily wanted me to meet Larry and get to know him. As
I told her about the other AIDS families with whom I was
involved, the tears of relief began to flow.

Emily was also deeply concerned for Larry's immediate
family, especially in relationship to the church. Since Larry
did not live in our community, the probability of their being
a part of our church family was remote. In fact, this was not
an issue at all as far as I was concerned. I assured her that
I would be happy to try to help them during this time of
grief and impending loss, in hopes that they would hear a
word from God as they walked through this dark valley.

Having been quietly rejected by his own church, Larry
had sought spiritual nurture in a church in Fort Lauderdale
that ministers primarily to the gay community. The pastor
and others in that church were crucial to Larry as he struggled with his impending death and validation as a person.
When Larry was finally unable to hold a full-time job, he
began working as a volunteer in the church and in the AIDS
center. He wanted badly to be able to give back something
to others who, like him, had overwhelming needs and were
dying.

Emily expressed a third concern that day. Larry's grandmother happened to be visiting at the time. The immediate
family had finally told the grandmother about Larry's illness. A deeply religious southern woman, she faced with

real bravery the fact that one of her grandsons was a homosexual and was dying with AIDS. Again, her deep faith and a strong family bond overrode questions about Larry's homosexuality. Larry was, after all, her grandson, and he was mortally ill. That was the important issue for her.

Larry wanted his grandmother to know about his situation, but he was uneasy about telling her. He felt that he would do so at a later time. He was not aware that she already knew. Emily now asked me if I would go with her to visit Larry's grandmother and discuss all this with her.

I gladly did so, and it was one of the most meaningful afternoons I have ever spent. Faced with such heavy news, along with the bleakness of her grandson's future, the grandmother still had a deep, abiding faith to see her and Larry through to the end, whenever that might be. I left the two women that afternoon with an overwhelming sense of the presence of the grace of God. Surely, God's grace is more than sufficient for all our needs.

This encounter was genuinely helpful for me as well. It underscored the need for an accepting love of persons even when there are things involved that we might not personally embrace or even fully understand. It served to strengthen my continuing commitment to make the issue of AIDS visible within our church. Surely, if in our small congregation four families were already dealing with this problem, there would be others in the months and years ahead. The more that people could know and understand, the better prepared they would be, as individuals—and we would be, as a church—to deal with what seemed inevitable.

The church must not ignore this problem or abandon the people involved. If ever there was a situation that needs the word and work of grace, it is the situation of those who are dealing with AIDS. The biblical revelation of God and the comfort of the Holy Spirit need to be shared especially in these kinds of situations. Throughout history, God has chosen the fragile vessels of people to be vehicles of grace and messengers of God's ministering presence and mercy. The fact that the nature of the disease called AIDS has some

troubling aspects to it, especially for the traditional ministry
of the church, does not excuse any of us from pretending
it is not there.

Shortly after my talk with Emily, I met Larry. He made a
point to come by the church for a visit. Frail and thin, he
wearily made his way up the steps to my office. After resting
a few minutes, he began to talk about where he was at this
point in his own personal journey.

On his own initiative, he shared with me his declaration
of his homosexuality as a teenager. He traced the pain and
suffering that made up that part of his life. The confusion
during his adolescence meant that there were long times of
deep depression. Attempts at ending his own life were a
part of the pain of his unfolding story. Among his most
difficult decisions was to confront his parents with his homosexuality.

Being an only child, he realized that there was no one else
to share in fulfilling the normal hopes and dreams of his
parents for grandchildren. Because of his homosexuality,
he experienced what he called a sense of failure on his part.
Even though his parents accepted him as a person and as
a son, the deeper question of personal failure was still
present in Larry's mind and heart.

His participation in the gay church in Fort Lauderdale
was a very special time in his life. Here was a community
that accepted him as he was. It was the only place he had
found where his homosexuality did not become a barrier to
ministry and development of his spiritual growth.

Whatever one's personal view and opinion of the "gay
church" might be, the sad fact is evident that they often
minister because others cannot or will not. Larry was honestly struggling with the relationship of his homosexuality
and his religion. He desperately wanted to know and understand what the scripture had to say. Because of his illness,
active sexuality was no longer an issue. As he faced death,
he needed above all to get his life right with God.

Interestingly enough, Larry was not looking for a minister or church just to say that being a homosexual was all

right and God really did not mind. As his illness progressed, he dealt with that very question as to whether it was right and could he be a Christian and a homosexual too. Larry admitted quite openly to me that it would have been much easier if he could have struggled with these issues in the church in which he grew up. As he said, "I would have loved to have gone back to where I first learned about God and the forgiveness of Christ to deal with what was happening to me." Unfortunately, that was not possible, so he went to the only place that seemed available to him.

Like Tom, Larry was at that place in his illness where he was dealing with closure. He wanted to make sure that all the loose ends of his life were tied up as neatly as possible. I was impressed that both Tom and Larry deeply wanted their lives to count for something. Both of them acknowledged that, if given another chance, their choices would be quite different. Neither of them wanted to die without feeling that their lives had counted for something, somewhere, somehow.

The pulling together of their stories, and what I as a pastor and we as a church learned together, had its birth in their wishes. I promised them both to do everything I could to continue to deal with AIDS as we encountered opportunities. I made a covenant to tell their stories, with the deep hope and prayer that others might learn something, both from their experiences and from those of us in the church. If the struggle of other AIDS patients and their families can be made a little easier, because their stories help other ministers and churches, their lives will not have been in vain.

2

The Minister's
Personal Preparation

Realization came early, in our journey with AIDS, that if I was going to continue to be a relevant and helpful pastor to Tom and Ruth and the others, I would need some preparation of my own.

The figures being used by the medical community to estimate the present and future numbers of our population that are and will be infected with the AIDS virus are staggering. From the present figure of 25,000 to 30,000 known cases in 1987,[2] the disease is expected to spread to include some 270,000 persons by the end of 1991.[3] That is only a few short years away.

These numbers mean that, without question, churches of all sizes and kinds will be touched by AIDS in increasing numbers. What is most alarming and depressing is that each number is a person who is probably going to die. These persons and their respective circles of family and friends stand in need of some form of ministry as they live with this harsh reality.

Even though we are located in one of the AIDS hot spots, the makeup of our church is much like hundreds and thousands of other suburban churches across the country. As AIDS spreads more and more into the heterosexual community, the issue of how churches like ours need to respond becomes more and more crucial.

Any time a new issue appears, it is tempting for ministers

to look for some how-to article on the subject. Another temptation is to seek out a similar situation for which a ministry has been developed and then try to duplicate that ministry in one's own setting. While this may work well for some persons in some situations, it will not work for the issue of AIDS.

While nearly all churches will be touched in one way or another by AIDS in the future, it will be the unusual church that has large numbers of patients for which a major program can be developed. Ministry to AIDS patients and their families cannot be handled through church programming, like food or clothing distribution or a specific age-group ministry.

The major thrust of any church's response to AIDS will be through pastoral caregivers, both lay and professional. The issue of confidentiality by itself almost precludes general lay involvement. The pastor will either do most of the ministry personally or will carefully build and train a group of lay people to assist. The crux of ministry to families dealing with AIDS inevitably revolves around the office of the pastor. Therefore, the pastor's investment of time for personal preparation is essential before any kind of ministry can happen in a given community.

Intellectual Preparation

My first step was to learn all I could about the disease itself. I began to read everything I could find in order to educate myself on the subject of the Acquired Immune Deficiency Syndrome. I started a file which has grown to be several files, divided according to their content. One file contains primarily medical information, reports, and articles. Most of these have a common element: data from the Centers for Disease Control in Atlanta, Georgia. I have found them helpful in working with AIDS patients and their families, and they have also enabled me to offer corrective and factual information in the many conversations where the subject of AIDS arises. This is especially true as people discuss how the disease is transmitted. By having current factual information at hand, it is possible to make a small contribution to dealing with AIDS hysteria.

Another file contains primarily news stories about AIDS and issues related to the disease. These have been the easiest to gather because there are so many of them. They are also the ones, however, that require the closest examination for bias and slant. A third file contains personal accounts of those dealing with AIDS. These often tragic stories have taught me a great deal about how to respond and how not to respond to those suffering with this disease.

My basic piece of educational material is the *Surgeon General's Report on Acquired Immune Deficiency Syndrome.* Published in October 1986, it is available on request from the U.S. Public Health Service in Washington, D.C. This report is clear and concise and is written in easy-to-understand language. It is dependable from a medical point of view and is, in my opinion, the single best piece of material available on the subject of the disease itself.

Much of my education has come from the medical community. Visits with doctors with whom Tom and Ruth had appointments proved to be an invaluable source of information. You might begin by discussing the disease with your own medical doctor. In addition, your local Public Health Service and American Red Cross office will have some very helpful material and persons to assist you. The American Red Cross has an excellent educational film that is available through local offices. Perhaps there is a visiting nurse association, hospice, or home health care service in your community. In all probability, these persons are already involved in the day-to-day care of AIDS patients; they can be of great help to any minister or church in their educational task. (See the Appendix for specific listings.)

In many large cities, the gay community will have some kind of formal group gathered to respond to those in their own locality who suffer from AIDS. There may be even a more formal AIDS center as such, established for the express purpose of responding to the disease. It was through our local AIDS center in Fort Lauderdale that I began to become more involved in the AIDS issue. As an outgrowth of going to support-group meetings with Tom and Ruth, I volunteered to visit and assist wherever possible from a pastoral perspective. We now have a Clergy Advisory Group made up of pastors from around the county in an effort to give some direction to the religious response within the community.

An excellent example of cooperation between the larger community and the pastoral community came after Christmas 1986, just before Larry died. One of the visiting nurses who was dealing with his case, knowing that I had been involved, called to tell me that Larry was in his final days of life. Her conversations with Larry had begun to deal with religious closure, and she felt I needed to respond personally to those issues. I thanked God for this sensitive nurse, who provided so much more than just basic nursing care. Her presence greatly enabled me to do my task, not only better but with a sense of encouragement that I was not alone in this business of AIDS ministry.

It is very important to learn as much as possible about this disease. This part of the journey was stimulating and challenging for me. However, it is important to remember that the skills we pastors already know and use daily are helpful too. Even as I was moving into new and unfamiliar territory, it was reassuring to be reminded that I already had some invaluable tools at my disposal.

There was one issue to which I had to be especially sensitive. This was the question of the focus of attention in terminal cases. In most such situations, little attention is given to how the disease occurred; the issue to be confronted is death itself, not its cause. However, with AIDS, some careful and sensitive pastoral attention and skill must be paid to the context in which the disease was contracted.

Since sexual activity is the major form of transmitting this disease, it is important to help the patient deal with this side of the issue. This can be both complicated and painful. For instance, many patients are facing the disclosure of lifestyles or habits that had previously been unknown. Often, family members are not involved with the patient until the disease has progressed significantly. Therefore, time becomes a valuable commodity.

Not only is there the fact of death to be faced, but often there are issues of anger, guilt, shame, or remorse to be worked through by both the patient and the family. This is especially poignant for those patients whose lifestyles have been recognized as unacceptable by most of society. Having felt rejection from the world in which they lived, the question of whether God, too, will reject them becomes an issue of paramount importance.

Involvement in these situations calls for learning all one can about the disease itself and the complexities involved in responding to it, as well as a careful reaffirmation of what one already knows about giving pastoral care. In dealing with AIDS patients and their families, there is no substitute for the minister's being intellectually prepared.

Emotional Preparation

I discovered, however, that intellectual preparation was only the beginning. There is also the task of being emotionally prepared. This part of the journey is the most difficult. It is possible to treat a given piece of information about AIDS in a fairly academic and impersonal way. But dealing with this material at the level of one's feelings is much harder. My own motivation did not come out of a deeply felt need for emotional growth. Quite frankly, it was my commitment to those persons in our church family with whom I was being called to minister that forced me to process what was going on inside.

Some of my early fears were related to the personal question of risk for me and my family. Even though I was told otherwise, I was still shaken a bit at the prospect, however irrational or slight, that I might be exposing myself and my family to a disease that, if contracted, would be fatal.

I was intellectually aware of what doctors at the University of Miami clinic and elsewhere were saying. I listened closely to my friend Kay, who also works at the medical school. I knew what I was supposed to believe. I knew the facts. Still, some unsettled fear was present, if I was honest enough to admit it. I began to dwell on the very small percentage of persons infected with AIDS who fall outside of all of the high-risk-behavior groups. While the medical experts do not agree on the exact percentage, they all agree that, for a very small number of AIDS cases, the source of infection has not been documented. My awareness of this number, however small, kept the fear alive and growing. Perhaps there are ways that AIDS can be contracted that the medical community just does not know about yet, I thought. In my more irrational moments, my fear even began to suggest to me that perhaps there are things they know and are not telling us.

It became apparent that, to be able to respond to Tom or Larry or anyone else I might encounter in ministry, I was going to have to deal with what I was feeling. I talked with my wife and children about the differences between what I knew and what I feared. I tried to keep a sense of balance. At the same time I wanted to be honest with them. My involvement with Tom and Larry and others meant that if there was any risk at all involved, my family would be exposed to the risk as well. Their response was serious but encouraging. They were grateful to be included in the discussion and not taken for granted. Then my son helped put things in perspective. He observed that from the facts and percentages I was sharing with them, there might be minimal risk involved. He also reminded me that there was risk involved in most of what we do, such as driving on I-95. His final statement was the clincher. He said, "Well, Dad, I guess it comes down to whether or not you think Tom and Ruth are worth the risk. Personally, I do. It really does not bother me to know that you are involved with people with AIDS." The brashness and indomitability of adolescence was obvious. Equally obvious was the biblical reality of being led by a child.

We agreed as a family that I had their blessing and that they were not overly concerned about my being involved. This "rite of passage" in my journey with AIDS helped me process this part of the emotional baggage that goes with it.

I was equally encouraged and a little surprised to discover that Kay and her husband had had a similar conversation. We were having one of those lunchtimes of mutual encouragement, and I shared with her my conversation with my family. She indicated with a smile that she had done the same thing with her husband. Even though she knew, intellectually, a great deal about AIDS, she too had to process the emotional side of her work.

To know I was not the only one who had some fears greatly helped relieve my feelings of guilt. Each time I had fears about myself and my family, I would feel guilty about not trusting the medical information we had been given. This guilt even raised the question of my trust in God. If indeed my ministry was calling me to deal with persons with AIDS, surely would not God protect me? Then I would get caught up in childhood memories of stories about a missionary, Lottie Moon, who went to China and died there of starvation because she gave her food to the children around her. I was not ready to be added to the list of martyrs who give their lives in sacrificial ministry. Martyrdom is easy to preach but difficult to practice.

I finally concluded that while there might be some risks, the facts were much more convincing. I also recalled that I had tried to work hard not to let other fears I had experienced control my life. This part of my life and ministry should be no exception. Fears, if left unchallenged, will grow to the point where one can truly get lost in them. I decided that facts and faith were strong partners and I would trust what I knew. Whatever risk was indeed present could be lived with.

The important issue is not where I came out but that I had to deal with this emotional aspect in my own preparation. Just working with people with AIDS and knowing some facts

without integrating them into what I was feeling would be
to miss the point and result in a ministry that would lack real
integrity.

Closely related to this part of my emotional trip was my
early fear that if others in the church found out I was ministering to AIDS patients, they would not want me around
them. I could be putting my ministry in jeopardy. My conversation with Dr. Dickinson at the clinic in Miami was
critical in my dealing with this. Working my way through
this fear has been a real help in remaining sensitive to
what others might feel about being involved with persons
with AIDS. This is especially true when others in the
church community raise this question. Having faced it myself enables me to hear at least some of what they are saying. In addition, dealing with this has given me a sense of
freedom to assume a leadership role within our congregation.

There is yet another dimension to the emotional side of
this journey. One cannot deal honestly with someone who
is terminally ill without at some point dealing with one's
own mortality. It is difficult to see others die, especially
young adults. It is much easier to talk about those parts of
our faith that deal with death than to have the experience.
Even though, from a religious perspective, we know about
the naturalness of death and all the promises of eternal life,
we are still brought up short when we really have to face the
fact that we will not live forever.

I found this particularly poignant with both Tom and
Larry. They certainly had to live with a different reality of
death than most of us do. As a result, they carefully reor-
dered their lives and their priorities. Life took on the dimensions of "gift" for them in ways that most of us take for
granted. Tom literally began to get his house in order with
each passing week. He was concerned that a new roof be put
on their home and that Ruth have more dependable trans-
portation before he died. He made sure a current will was
drawn up. One of the most painful parts was our visit with
the local funeral director to make burial arrangements. It

was important to Tom to arrange all this himself so Ruth would not have to deal with the details. He needed to care for some of these kinds of concerns so that the time he had could be quality time for him and Ruth.

I was especially touched by the approach that Larry made to Christmas in 1986, which was his last. It was his intent, I believe, to hold on to life until Christmas. He wanted his last Christmas to be good. Shopping was a physical impossibility for him. However, he was very concerned that the right gifts be bought for his family. A good friend suggested that he go and purchase several items and bring them to the house for Larry to look at and to choose from. Those not chosen would simply be returned. This way Larry was able to do his "Christmas shopping" and have the assurance that his parents, whom he loved so dearly, would have just the right gift from him.

Walking with Tom and Larry through these experiences was deeply moving. How easy it is to take the gift of life lightly! We think we have all the time in the world to get things done. Walking alongside of death, especially with those who are near to us and close to our age, has a strange way of reminding us of our own mortality. While this was a painful reality at times, it also helped me reassess my own values and priorities.

There is another dimension to the death issue for the minister of those with AIDS. The present medical reality is that there is no cure for AIDS. It is ultimately 100 percent fatal. Therefore, from the very outset of ministry, with either a person with AIDS or a family member, the reality is that unless something intervenes we do not yet know about, this person will die. It is very depressing to know the score before the game is over.

This is a real issue with AIDS patients themselves. There seems to be an incredibly tight network among them. They know when someone is sick again and how bad it looks. Word about recent funerals always spreads quickly. In the two years that Tom had AIDS, he saw about twenty-five people die that he had encountered one way or another in the AIDS network. If it is difficult for me, I would think, what must that reality be doing to him?

There is also a ripple effect out into the community at large, especially among those people who are participating in high-risk behavior but do not yet have the disease. I have talked with many people about the intense fear they live with each day, knowing what the possibilities are. For some, the fear has been sufficient to cause a change in behavior. For others, the behavior continues and the fear heightens each day. Probably there are folks like this sitting in nearly every church on Sunday, trying to deal with these kinds of feelings.

At a funeral I conducted for an AIDS patient, I was deeply moved by the faces of some of those in attendance. The patient himself had been very visible in the gay community, and many of his friends were present. I had met some of them before. As the service progressed, the tension and fear about whose funeral would be next was so obvious on their faces, I could not help feeling my own pain for the load they must carry each day of their lives.

As long as there is no cure for AIDS, this issue will need to be faced by everyone in touch with these patients. One hopes there will be enough pastoral care to make a difference.

Perhaps the most surprising part of examining the emotional side of my own ministry with AIDS patients and their families came from having to deal with people whose lifestyles lie outside the realm of my own experience and that of most church communities.

Getting involved with Tom and Ruth as they began their journey into the world of AIDS, I began to notice some unusual feelings. Given the reality that about 70 percent of those persons suffering with AIDS are in the homosexual or bisexual communities,[4] it was inevitable that the three of us would be thrown into this world as well. The meetings available to AIDS patients, sponsored by the AIDS centers in Fort Lauderdale and Miami, were mainly attended by gay men. Tom, especially, began to feel some discomfort. This straight street-wise crane operator was very conscious of the ways that he and his experiences were different from most of the others in the support group.

The groups provide a valuable place for AIDS patients to gather and share mutual concerns and fears and to draw support from each other. Tom tried groups in both Fort Lauderdale and Miami. They all had a professional there to help lead the group and keep dialogue from getting bogged down. Tom, Ruth, and I all talked on more than one occa-sion about needing to get past our own concerns of being in a group of primarily gay people before much real help could be gained. There were times that Tom's level of dis-comfort was so high he chose not to participate in the meet-ings.

As an outgrowth of attending these groups, I decided to provide pastoral ministry to others who did not have access to such help, so I went to a training session for volunteers conducted by the Fort Lauderdale AIDS center. The meet-ing took place on a Saturday morning at one of the local hotels on the beach. As one of the main hotels that catered to gay tourists, it was fairly well known as the "gay hotel" by most local residents. The meeting was helpful and the time was well spent. As I left the hotel and walked out of the front door to my car, however, I was thinking, Now, how would I explain to someone who saw me coming out of the gay hotel on the beach, midday on a Saturday, just what I was doing there in the first place? I kind of chuckled to myself about the question, but it stayed with me nonethe-less.

Any visible identity that I had with the AIDS community would inevitably mean that I would be consistently around and involved in groups of gay people. That involvement had hardly been a part of my regular pattern as pastor of First Baptist Church, out in the quiet, "safe" suburb of Plantation. Here was another risk that had to be assessed. This time, it was neither my health nor my vocational identity that was the issue. Now, the risk focused on my identity as a person—as a male—as I would be viewed through the eyes of other people.

Pastoral Preparation

As I lived with this quiet concern, I found I was not only dealing with an emotional, psychological issue but with a biblical one as well. Association and identity with individuals and groups of people were only part of the issue. The biblical injunction to be present in the name of Christ with the cup of cold water, the visits, the involvement with those in need, regardless of their identity or lifestyle, was abundantly clear. The searching question of Jesus as recorded in the twenty-fifth chapter of Matthew's gospel remained before me: Where were you when I was hungry, thirsty, a stranger, naked, sick, and in prison? AIDS people were certainly sick, and definitely strangers! To let a decision of my involvement with AIDS patients be influenced by my own uneasiness, or by my fears of what conclusions others would draw, left me far short of being able to answer Jesus' question. Living with the identity drawn from pastoring a typical suburban church was easy. Expanding that identity to include pastoring people with AIDS was another thing entirely.

I had to recognize that my identity was important, but only in the context of ministering to people, whoever they were or however strange their lifestyle. The more I lived with the model of Jesus himself, the easier this issue became for me. If Jesus was indeed an example for us by going through Samaria (see John 4) rather than going around, as was the traditional route for the devout Jew, it seemed that as his disciple I could do no less. It would indeed be easier in many respects to go around those places and those people involved with AIDS than it would to go to where they were and become involved with them. In fact, Jesus seemed to go out of his way to meet those who had been overlooked—or literally "looked over"—or labeled or cast aside by society. The trip through Samaria is just one of many examples in the life and ministry of Jesus that illustrate this point. His ministry consistently took him into the lives of tax collectors, publicans, lepers, prostitutes, the poor, the dispossessed, and crowds of others whom tradition and religion had not only cast aside but labeled "less than."

This recognition came painfully and slowly for me. After all, my full-time task was pastoring a church in a community that was quite different from that in which the majority of the AIDS patients live. But the reality was that AIDS had indeed come to our church.

It was several months before I referred to AIDS and my involvement with it in a sermon. Each time I made such a reference, I watched and listened closely to the response from the church. *There was never, to my knowledge, a negative reaction.* If anything, there was a response of gratitude on the part of the congregation that I, on behalf of our religious community, was present and involved.

I have now made numerous references in sermons to the issue of AIDS as well as to my own involvement. Sometimes the reference was to my involvement with those in our own church family. Other times, the mention was related to my work with those in the larger community who were dying with AIDS and had no other pastoral resources.

The congregational response, along with other indications of support, really helped to confirm my decision to be involved in whatever way I can, wherever that takes me. From this vantage point, after almost three years of involvement, it is easy to look back and wonder why I spent so much time worrying. However, when I was faced with questions at the beginning of this journey, they were very important to me. There is no way to underscore the importance of working through all the questions that arise in ministry to people with AIDS.

Any pastor already knows the importance of confidentiality in the everyday task of pastoral care. In pastoral ministry, confidentiality spells credibility. Without it, the pastor's work is rendered almost ineffective.

I had learned with Ruth and Tom that, especially in the world of AIDS, confidentiality is perhaps the most difficult and sensitive area. It is not uncommon for AIDS victims to lose their jobs and find themselves, when disclosed as having AIDS, not only unemployed but also without any medical insurance. Others find that their normal support community disappears. Still others find that even their own families cannot deal with their having AIDS and quietly withdraw their support and presence as well.

In addition, I was aware of some pitfalls in regard to AIDS and the issue of confidentiality. In another church, a member who contracted AIDS told his pastor about his situation. In trying to be redemptive and supportive, the pastor shared this knowledge with the congregation so they could support this particular church member during the most serious crisis of his life. The result was that this man lost his job when his employer discovered that he had AIDS. In response, the AIDS patient sued the church and the minister. It is unbelievable how quickly problems concerning AIDS can multiply. Sensitivity to these issues is a must if we are going to minister effectively.

It therefore becomes necessary sometimes not to disclose all you know about a person's illness. This is especially true in the early stages of the disease, when some normal activity can still take place. Many AIDS patients are able to function and hold their jobs for several months following diagnosis.

For example, in Tom's case, after his diagnosis, he was still able to work and in fact needed to work for his own emotional health as well as for continued income and benefits. I have already explained how Tom and Ruth and I agreed not to disclose the exact nature of Tom's illness until he became unable to work and the problem of loss of job no longer was an issue. There was also the very real question of job security for Ruth. She might well be out of a job, should her employer discover that her husband had AIDS.

As long as it was just the three of us talking about it, confidentiality posed no real problem. However, as Tom was in and out of the hospital repeatedly, the normal concern of our community surfaced. As a church, we have prided ourselves on the integrity of the level of caring we have for one another in our family of faith. Our church ministry seemed strongest when a time of crisis would arrive in the lives of one of our families. We were accustomed to dealing factually with one another about what was happening in our midst as a way to ensure honest ministry.

The questions from church members who really cared about Tom as a friend and church member became more difficult to answer as his illness progressed. The questions were concerned ones from people who loved and cared about Tom and Ruth. Not being able to deal openly with them was a problem.

When asked "What is really wrong with Tom?" I learned to reply with partial information, and for the most part that was sufficient. Several of the more well read and perceptive people recognized the symptoms and realized what was happening. Many simply concluded that Tom had some kind of cancer. As his condition weakened and his attendance at church became more irregular, the questions persisted. I was especially sensitive to them when Tom and Ruth did come to church, because his illness was very visible in his tremendous weight loss.

Confidentiality in this situation and in these circumstances meant protection from unemployment and consequent loss of insurance for as long as possible. And there was another dimension: This was Tom and Ruth's story to tell, not mine. It was his body that was being destroyed, their lives that were being turned upside down. There was no real alternative but to respect their wishes and be supportive of their position. I would just have to sidestep questions until circumstances allowed a full disclosure.

Such a time came for Tom all too soon. His hospitalization in December 1985 for a serious bout with *Pneumocystis carinii* pneumonia made him unable to return to work. Not only did Tom then deal with his work situation, but we were able to answer more completely the questions that would come. In one sense it was a relief to be totally open with church members regarding these two people and their upside-down lives. In another, more painful sense, it was quite difficult because to be able to speak frankly meant that Tom was moving that much closer to death.

Thank God we have progressed in society a bit, in that job loss just due to identification of AIDS is happening less and less. A recent lawsuit filed in Fort Lauderdale by a Broward County employee, Todd Shuttleworth, who was dismissed because of AIDS, resulted in his being reinstated in his job and given back pay.[5] What is being referred to as the "Shuttleworth decision" may become a benchmark in the issue of litigation and confidentiality in the world of AIDS.

Even though job security may become less and less of an issue, the very real issue of relationships to co-workers, friends, neighbors, and family members still remains. I encountered the relationship side of the confidentiality issue in the death of Larry. I was aware that Larry's immediate family were fully aware both of his homosexuality and of his having AIDS. In fact, the response of Larry's family will always stand in my mind as a magnificent demonstration of love that knows no bounds. Like Tom and Ruth, they too dealt with the reality that only those immediately connected to the family needed to know the details. Family members who lived away and were not part of the day-to-day developments remained, by family decision, uninformed of all the facts.

On the night before Larry's funeral, the pain of the confidentiality issue became very clear to me. I was sitting in the living room with his parents, planning the service to be held the next day. It was important that we do this painful task together. Larry had talked to several of us at different times about what he wanted at his funeral. We needed to compare notes in order to be able to carry out Larry's wishes. It was also important to me that his parents wanted—indeed, needed to have—their own input into the exact nature of the service. Even though we all wanted to respect Larry's wishes, it was his parents who would have to live with the

memory of the funeral service. Both as the officiating minister and as their friend, I needed the assurance that they
were comfortable with the basic direction of the service.
They had experienced an immense amount of pain in the
past few years. I wanted the service to be a strengthening
time for them, a real prelude to healing.

Larry's mother was very concerned about any reference
that I might make to why Larry had died. Through tears, she
explained painfully that their decision not to share everything with the whole family may not have been the right
one. But the funeral was hardly the time to break the news
that Larry was gay and died with AIDS. We agreed that
confidentiality would be continued in this situation even
after death.

There is no way to describe the depth of suffering I observed in these loving, grieving parents. The loss of an only
child at age twenty-seven was painful enough. The decision
not to share the details and circumstances only compounded it.

This issue figured significantly in their decision as to the
kind of service we would have. They had long respected
Larry's need to be a part of the gay church community in
Fort Lauderdale. They talked between themselves as to
whether to have the service in Larry's church or in a more
traditional one. The choice was made to have a traditional
setting.

On the day of the funeral I looked out at family members
who had come to the service and who loved Larry, yet due
to the issue of confidentiality they did not know the whole
story that figured so heavily into the pain and grieving of his
parents. In addition, in the church that afternoon sat two of
the ministers from the gay community who had ministered
so significantly to Larry when other more "traditional" ministers not only refused but in essence had withdrawn fellowship from him. I had spent enough time talking with Larry
in the last six months of his life to know that much of the
spiritual peace he began to experience came as a result of
their involvement with him. The need for continued confi-

dentiality meant that they could only sit quietly along with other friends and family during the funeral service, even though Larry's parents were deeply grateful for the ministry of all of the people who touched Larry's life, including those in the gay community.

The issue of confidentiality in the world of AIDS can take on unique and unexpected dimensions. That it demands and deserves the critical attention of the ministering community cannot be overemphasized.

Another aspect of AIDS may also raise significant questions. Unlike other diseases, AIDS is generally associated with behavior that is not acceptable to a large percentage of our population. Many diseases that result in death have their beginnings in behavior. Smoking has been linked to lung cancer, alcohol to liver disease, and improper diet—especially in the area of cholesterol—to heart disease. We have long been familiar with the relationship between certain kinds of "high-risk behavior" and the illnesses and diseases that often result. However, the major difference between the foregoing list and the behavior associated with homosexuality and drug use is that smoking, drinking, overeating, and improper diet have all become acceptable.

Behaviors associated with homosexual or bisexual persons and I.V. drug users have been medically identified as very high-risk behaviors in relation to AIDS. But these behaviors would not be called acceptable by a broad section of our population. This often results in participation in these areas being kept secret, or "in the closet," as the popular phrase puts it.

Many people function in the closet for years and years. It is not uncommon for people to live a whole lifetime in this fashion. Often they die, from other causes besides AIDS, without even those closest to them ever discovering the hidden side of their lives.

But when AIDS comes into the picture the patient's lifestyle will eventually become fairly apparent. The medical community is doing an excellent job in communicating to the general public that AIDS is almost always transmitted through sexual or drug-related activities. Disclosure becomes inevitable for the vast majority of those contracting the disease.

For those persons who take seriously their ministry to people with AIDS, the question of lifestyle becomes a major issue. The difficult and often painful task of helping people through AIDS as a terminal illness is demanding and complex in itself. When another dimension is added, that of disclosing the lifestyle through which the disease was contracted, the problem is compounded.

This double effect is an issue in many cases now. As AIDS continues to spread into the heterosexual community, especially through bisexual, adulterous, or promiscuous activities, it will become more and more of a major concern with which we must deal. Ministering persons who are called upon to share in the lives of people with AIDS will often find themselves dealing with the grief of facing terminal illness and, at the same time, the shock and surprise of a lifestyle heretofore unrevealed to friends and relatives.

I am working now with a family that is confronting this problem. The father has AIDS. He and his wife had separated before he became ill: his wife, already concerned about his use of cocaine, had begun to have suspicions about his sexuality. The situation became such that she decided she and the children needed to leave. It was sometime following this separation that the diagnosis of AIDS was confirmed—which also confirmed his heretofore hidden bisexuality.

Now she is dealing with the imminent death of someone she loves as well as having to internalize the fact that he was bisexual as well. She is also dealing with what to tell the children. At this point, they believe he got AIDS from drugs, and she considers this to be sufficient. It is an incredibly complex situation. Walking with them through this experience takes a great deal of care and an immense amount of energy. I keep at it because the reality with which I am struggling is minimal in relation to what they are dealing with.

As a pastor, I find a great deal of strength from the experience of Jesus with the Samaritan woman at Jacob's well (John 4). I keep going back to this story because there are several very interesting things about it in the context of dealing with AIDS from a pastoral perspective.

First of all, this encounter involved a person who was both a Samaritan and a woman. If Jesus was making any kind of point to his followers about dealing with those different from the establishment, he scored a double hit by the setting and person involved.

Second, it was Jesus who brought about the disclosure, who led the conversation into uncovering who the woman really was. The woman from Sychar only responded to his leadership. Surely, if Jesus himself was not afraid of dealing with this information, I as a pastor can risk being present when the facts about a lifestyle become known. I do not need to fear either the disclosure or the complications that result, for they both provide the context for ministry.

Third, it was after her situation was revealed that the woman from Sychar encountered the full impact of who Jesus was. As painful and complex and even embarrassing as disclosure might be, it is only at that point that any kind of honest response to the presence of God could take place. Disclosure made honesty possible. Likewise, for us, there is a powerful relationship between disclosure, honesty, and the presence of God.

It would be great if our personal preparation to confront AIDS could be completed once and for all. However, such is not the case. The need is constantly changing as we change. We discover new truths about ourselves, and these insights have to be related to the situations we encounter in ministry. As difficult and lonely as some of this part of the journey has been for me personally, I am nonetheless growing more deeply aware that if I will risk ministry, God's grace is more than sufficient for all my needs.

3

The Minister's Theological Preparation

When AIDS does come to church, it becomes our turn to respond, and the question of how we will respond becomes paramount. By the very nature of who the church is as the people of God, our response will be a theological one. What we believe about God as Creator and Sustainer will mold our answer.

Judgment or Compassion?

In the relatively short time since AIDS was reported in our society—1981—[6] we can already see how theology has shaped the response of the church. Some ministers, in addressing both the issue of AIDS and the individuals infected with the virus, have responded from a viewpoint of judgmental theology; their statements have almost always included some clear word of judgment, spoken by the church on God's behalf, to those who are suffering with this disease. The presence of AIDS, both in society and in individuals, is seen as clear evidence of the wrathful judgment of God in reply to the behavior that caused the disease to be contracted.

Some of those who choose to respond out of a judgmental theology have even gone to the extreme of implying that God created AIDS specifically for the purpose of punishing certain groups in society. The two groups most singled out by this approach, of course, are in the gay and drug communities. The response from a judgmental theology centers on the difference between those who have AIDS and those who do not. Separateness is its main focus. Further, it seems to use AIDS to dramatize the power of God's judgment; the presence of a terminal illness in a person's life becomes a platform for proclaiming the judgment of God. This response also points out the consequences for those who make the kinds of choices that can result in contracting the disease.

There is also a prophetic response in judgmental theology. Often the existence of the disease is used to call for changes in the way people live. This response seeks to speak clearly to what can happen in the lives of individuals and in society at large unless changes in lifestyles occur.

There is a second approach, which can be identified as coming from an incarnational theology. This approach focuses on creating a presence on behalf of God in the lives of those dealing with AIDS. Issues such as acceptance, affirmation, and belonging are paramount.

In contrast to judgmental theology, a response out of an incarnational theology is based on the similarities that we have with those who have AIDS. It focuses on the ways we are alike in our capacity, as creations of God, to make some of the same choices that others have made in contracting AIDS. It amplifies that part of our creation that says we need each other, especially in times of crisis. It builds its response out of a deep and unsettling awareness that "there, but for the grace of God, go I." An incarnational response centers on the people who are dying rather than on how they became ill. It struggles with a way to be present in their lives as the incarnate Word of God. An incarnational response understands the biblical reality that we are indeed our "brother's brother and our sister's sister," and their keeper as well.

Recognizing the existence of these two general responses by the church raises another important factor—our need to learn to differentiate between the various ways that the disease can be contracted. Because AIDS surfaced in this country primarily in the homosexual community, it has mistakenly been identified as a "gay disease." AIDS is not a gay disease. Research and statistics show that, worldwide, AIDS is clearly a heterosexual disease. AIDS is most often—not always—sexually transmitted. Medical experts tell us that this will come to be the case in our society also, as the disease spreads. There is no question that the largest number of AIDS patients at the present time have contracted the disease through homosexual activity. Second to these patients are those who contracted the disease through I.V. drug use. These are followed by those who have been identified as "innocent victims"—those persons who contracted the disease through blood transfusions or who are spouses of AIDS patients and contracted the disease through normal sexual activity with husband or wife before knowledge of the presence of the disease surfaced. Perhaps the most "innocent" of all are those children born with the disease because the mother was infected during the pregnancy.

Understandably, it is easier to respond to those who are the most innocent. Visiting at Jackson Memorial Hospital in Miami, I encountered a beautiful little girl who was about two years old. The chaplain pointed out that she had AIDS. Her face and arms already bore the telltale marks of Kaposi's sarcoma, the cancer that is often associated with AIDS. Any feeling person would be immediately moved with compassion for this child. However, had the patient been twenty-nine years old and a gay male, the response might be quite different.

We are called by God to exercise discernment, the capacity to distinguish between things that differ (1 Cor. 12:10). Unless we learn to differentiate, we can easily lose sight of people as we respond. We must not operate on a theological conclusion based on the assumption that AIDS is simply a gay disease and is God's punishment to that particular group of people. We must be very careful to distinguish between the different ways the disease can be contracted. We must let our skill in differentiating help us focus on the fact that persons with AIDS are people who are dying. Some of them have contracted the disease through such sexual activity as homosexuality, bisexuality, adultery, or promiscuity. No matter. We must be careful to focus on people and not fall into the tempting trap of identifying them by groups and responding to that identity. Granted, it is much easier to let our theology focus on labeling people than it is to let our theology move us into authentic biblical ministry. We must not let labels determine our ministry.

The medical community is already dealing with this very issue. Early in their study of this disease, one heard and read a lot about high-risk "groups." The concern of contracting the disease focused on what kind of group you belonged to: homosexual, bisexual, I.V. drug user, and so on. There is now a healthy shift in the literature and communication. The medical community is talking about high-risk "behavior" instead of high-risk "groups." The riskiest behavior is promiscuity of any kind. If we focus on the behavior, perhaps it will be easier to see AIDS patients as people with various needs and lifestyles. The emphasis shifts from how people contract the disease to the fact that they have it.

The church does not need to abandon its prophetic role in society. It does not need to abdicate its concern with lifestyle choices and behaviors which result in people becoming less than God intended for them. However, as we struggle with this, the biblical record is clear that our identity is as ministers of reconciliation. The apostle Paul clearly underscores in Romans that it is because of the "reconciling" work of God in Christ Jesus toward us that we are able to be God's children. The task of reconciliation by God is boldly seen in the coming of God in the person of Christ into our world in order to identify with us. Christ became one of us in order for us to know who God is. In Christ, God accepts us as we are with all our sins and shortcomings, whatever their nature. Out of that relationship of acceptance, Christ then calls us to belong to him and live for him.

Paul carries this same theme over into his letter to the

church at Corinth and indicates that we have been given the "ministry of reconciliation" (2 Cor. 5:18–19). The process then becomes obvious. Our task as we minister is to be able to accept people where they are, regardless of their label or identification. It is then, beginning with acceptance, that the process of reconciliation can even be possible.

Granted, we walk a fine line responding to persons with AIDS. We must neither condemn nor condone. Both attitudes are deadly. What we must do is seek to love and respond to the needs of people in the ways that God showed us in the person of Jesus Christ.

Ministry by labeling or ministry from labeling is a form of theological behavior which carries its own "high risk": that whole groups of people in our society will fall outside the reach of the church. To remain overly preoccupied with the issue of labels is to lose the ability to differentiate. Because there are so many others besides homosexuals and addicts who will contract this disease, and as predictions from the medical community become a reality and more heterosexual AIDS patients are diagnosed, this task should become somewhat clearer for the church. At that point we will have to deal with the presence and effects of this disease from a much broader and deeper perspective.

Perhaps it is so easy for some to consider AIDS a "gay disease" because of the current statistics. It is even understandable for some to relegate the disease to the "gays" and "druggies," groups with whom most of us do not have day-to-day contact. However, the whole scene will probably change when people in the heterosexual community begin to contract the disease in increasing numbers. After all, churches are not accustomed to having to deal with members dying from adultery or promiscuity. With the seemingly inevitable spread of this disease, the issue will suddenly belong to all of us in a whole new way.

When AIDS comes to church, we have to deal with the theological assumptions that undergird our response. Such preparation can and should be undertaken before AIDS actually arrives among us. Trying to be prepared before the fact will make the task of ministry much clearer and more manageable.

Created for Community and Responsibility

There are two broad theological issues in the context of the need to minister to persons with AIDS. The first issue, discussed in this chapter, has to do with our theological understanding of creation. The second issue, discussed in the next chapter, will deal with our understanding of the person, work, and ministry of Jesus as a model and example.

The biblical revelation from its very beginning in the book of Genesis tells us that the creation of humankind was different from all the other creatures God made. The portrait of creation in Genesis 1 and 2 shows a loving God molding and making man and woman and then gently blowing into them the breath of life. We have been made by God, and we bear God's mark upon us. The scripture says we were made in the image of God (Gen. 1:26–27). This means that there is a binding kind of relationship between us as God's creations, even though each of us is different and unique. The English poet John Donne said it well when he wrote those now-familiar words, "No man is an island, entire of itself; every man . . . is a part of the main." It is the very fact that we all bear the mark of the One who made us that binds us together.

Yet, at the same time, God has made us responsible for the gift of life and for the gift of this world in which we live. Unquestionably we are accountable to God for what we do with what God has given us. For those dealing with AIDS, that accountability comes stalking them in the person of death. AIDS can bring about death in a relatively short time. Or dying can also be a long-drawn-out affair. AIDS patients are almost without exception preoccupied with facing death. This is not necessarily the same as being afraid to die. It does mean that there is more often than not a deep concern with getting things in order before one meets the Maker.

Some of Larry's most painful and yet poignant moments before his death were concerned with this very issue. During his last hospitalization in early December of 1986, Larry found it necessary to look back through some of his life's experiences as a way of recounting for himself just where his journey had taken him. While talking was physically quite difficult at that point in his illness, he nonetheless made the effort to retrace his steps. He was dealing with the issue of accountability for what he had done with God's gift of life to him. While doing so was physically draining and emotionally painful for him, it needed to be done. I was confident that when Larry died several weeks later, just after Christmas, he had gotten his house in order. He had dealt with his personal relationship to God in Jesus Christ. He had had his time of confession. He had reaffirmed his own faith and belief as a child of God. He had reaffirmed his love and gratitude to his parents and close friends. He had done everything he could do and needed to do in order to face death.

For those of us who do not have AIDS and may never have AIDS, the issues of belonging to one another and of accountability are none the less present. As ministers of reconciliation, we will also be held accountable for the way we use the gift of life that God has given to us. One of the clearest pictures of that time called "judgment" is seen in the twenty-fifth chapter of Matthew in the New Testament. Jesus describes the final gathering as a time of separation between those who will spend eternity with God and those who will not. Interestingly enough, the separation will come as a response is given to the question from Jesus, Where were you when I was hungry, and naked, and sick, and in prison, and a stranger?

The issue of accountability of our stewardship of life as a gift from God is universal in its application. Understanding—both of the nature of our creation as made in the image of God and of our accountability for that very gift—is essential if we hope to provide ministry to those with AIDS and their families.

God not only made us in his image as responsible people finally accountable to him, God also made us as social creatures. Another way of saying this is that God did not create humankind to live in isolation. Again, the Genesis story sets the stage. When God made man, he went another step in deciding that it was not good for man to be alone (Gen. 2:18). Therefore, he made woman as a partner, a "helper" for him. Throughout the biblical record and down through history, the story of humankind's struggle with relationships unfolds. In the midst of all of the strengths and weaknesses revealed in that struggle is the outstanding idea that God did not make us to exist in isolation.

Nowhere is community more important than in a time of personal crisis. It is then that the child in all of us comes out regardless of our age and we feel a need to be noticed and held and taken care of. There can be few things worse during such times than being left alone or abandoned. Unfortunately, this becomes a real issue when AIDS comes into a person's life. I have been in tiny efficiency apartments where persons with AIDS have gone to die because their families and friends have cut them off, left them alone, out of fear or prejudice or whatever. One young man in a small one-room apartment had lost his job and also his insurance. He had nowhere else to go. When his family found out he was gay, they shut him out. His friends were confused and afraid to come around. He had kept his homosexuality a secret throughout his life, and now he was dying with AIDS. He was running out of money. He was running out of time. Worst of all, he had run out of friends and was alone. Being ill with AIDS had deprived him of one of the most basic needs given by God at creation, that of interaction with others. When I called back several days later, the apartment was empty and he was gone. I do not know to this day whether he died or whether someone finally came and began caring for him. My overwhelming memory is of this man, a child of God, alone.

The fear of isolation is very real among persons with AIDS. Many people pull back from those with AIDS because they are uninformed about how the disease can be transmitted. Some are informed but not sure they can trust what the medical community is saying. They, too, pull away. Others back off out of hurt and confusion over discovering a lifestyle that heretofore was hidden.

One AIDS patient spoke to this fear quite pointedly. He had learned that one of the nurses on the floor where he was hospitalized had been keeping visitors from seeing him. Because his immune system was not functioning, she felt he was at risk of being infected by people coming into his room. When he learned this, he let it be known that he was not in the least afraid to die, but he was terrified of being abandoned and isolated while he was dying. Even if others coming into his room meant infection of some sort for him, he was willing to risk that rather than suffer the pain of total isolation from other human beings.

It is imperative to remember our deep God-given need for community and relationship. Even though the biblical record and our own experience point out that we do not always do so well with our relationships with others, we certainly cannot do without them. Social interaction, not isolation, is part of the creation package.

When AIDS comes into the church itself, this issue becomes very real. Even though the presence of AIDS is handled in a confidential way, it is likely that those who are ill will fear isolation anyway. As Tom said, early in his illness, before the church in general knew of his disease, "My greatest fear is that I will lose the church when they find out I have AIDS." Since he was a new Christian, church was a form of life itself that he had not known before. His natural God-given need for community and human interaction was made more complex by the fact that the church was so very important to him. To deal with the possibility of having to face the last days of one's life alone and in isolation would be bad enough. To have to do so without those you love and care about would be almost unthinkable.

Theologically, we have been created by God, and we bear

the mark of God's image. We have been created as unique and special individuals who were made for interaction and community. We were not created for isolation. A part of our creation is bearing the responsibility and accountability to God for the gift of life to us. This is yet another side to our theology of creation that has real bearing on the issue of the response of the church to AIDS.

At the core of our creation is the gift of responsiveness from God. We have been created to love God, serve God, and live in warm fellowship with God. This responsiveness as a part of our creation is very significant. God has not made us and then capriciously cast us out into this world to make it the best way we can. We have not been abandoned by the One who made us.

Throughout the biblical revelation, we constantly see God moving toward humankind in an effort to relate to people and call them into relationship. The calling out of Abraham from Haran (Gen. 12:4) is one of the earliest reminders of this part of creation. God also called Moses out to gather up his people and lead them from slavery and bondage into new life as a special nation (Exodus 3 and 4). Illustrations abound in the Old Testament of God constantly moving toward humankind, working through the gift of freedom of will to connect with that responsive note implanted within us at creation.

Of course, the most dramatic evidence of this is the incarnation itself. God came in human form in the person of Jesus Christ to call us to God in the clearest and boldest way. Christ spent his ministry reaching for the responsiveness of humankind through all kinds of ways. Through the ministry of presence, of healing, of feeding, of touching, of forgiving, Christ directed himself toward that responsive chord in us. In preparation for his leaving this earth, Christ then gave to us the promise of the Holy Spirit, the comforter (John 14:16 KJV). The description of the Holy Spirit as the "comforter" who functions in the physical absence of Christ is itself a strong biblical basis for ministry to those with AIDS. We need to struggle honestly to embody the comforting nature of the Holy Spirit in all that we do in ministry.

The central task of discipling given to the church by Christ (Matt. 28:19–20) is based theologically on this issue of responsiveness. We cannot allow the presence of AIDS to be a barrier in carrying out this part of the ministry of the church. AIDS notwithstanding, we must continue to find ways to reach toward that responsiveness that is there as a part of our creation. There is a danger here to oversimplify and say that all God's creations are seeking ways to respond to God. This simply is not true. It is not even true of all AIDS patients.

Perhaps the clearest biblical example to illustrate this is found in the fifteenth chapter of Luke's Gospel, the story that has been called the Prodigal Son. It is easy, unless you are an "elder brother," to understand the reason the father threw such a party at his son's return. The younger son had taken his inheritance and squandered it. He made lifestyle choices that were far from what he had been raised to be and do. However, the younger son came to himself and decided to return home, even if he had to do so as a hired servant. The key to the story is the presence of the father. While the son was yet a long way off, he was spotted by the father, who began to celebrate. The father ran to him and hugged and kissed him before one word of confession was uttered. His presence and his actions said, I love you. I prize you. I welcome you home. After this emotional scene had taken place, words of confession came forth from the son.

Perhaps it would be a helpful exercise to recast this parable in the context of AIDS. Suppose the story had been different and the younger son came to himself because he discovered he had contracted AIDS while living it up in a far country. Suppose the confession had been a little different, something like, "Dad, I've come home because I have AIDS. I lost my job and my insurance, and I have come home to die." The central question again focuses on the response of the father. Given all the supporting biblical evidence of the nature of God, I believe the father's response would have been much the same; he still would have embraced him and welcomed him home. While the kind of party they had might have been different, there would have been celebration that, for whatever time was left, father and son would share it together. Of course, there would still be the elder brother, who perhaps will never understand why people like his brother should be welcomed home with such warmth and love, having lived the kind of life that resulted in AIDS. Viewing life from such a posture of self-righteousness nearly always causes people to miss the real point.

The real point is seen clearly in Luke's account of this parable and also in my contemporary version. The major issue is not the content of people's lives, not what they did in terms of specific activity. It is that a person who has lived very far from us and perhaps very differently from us has come into our presence. The model of the father in this parable underscores that the nature of God is constantly to reach toward that responsive chord deep within all of us. The church needs to learn how to embody the person of the Father and embrace all who come our way.

In the case of both Larry and Tom, the presence of their own families had a great deal to do with their ability to deal effectively with life. Several years before he contracted AIDS, Larry had decided that he needed to be open with his family about his homosexuality. Obviously, that was not an easy time for them. Both parents have said to me that, in the midst of those painful days, the reality kept surfacing that Larry was still their son, regardless of his sexual identity. That reality created a bond between them that carried them through the dark days of AIDS. I have never seen a more beautiful expression of "welcoming one home" than was evidenced by Larry's parents during his illness. Their acceptance, love, and nurture were present up to the night he died. They caught the point of this parable in Luke, and Larry certainly benefited. He could deal with whatever came his way.

Likewise, Tom was fortunate to have a wife like Ruth, who

chose to stand by him even though she disagreed with some of the things he did. When she was called upon to walk with him through AIDS, she could have done what other spouses and families have done; she could have left in fear or anger or just confusion and frustration. Ruth's situation is even more complex than that of Larry's parents, in that there is the very real risk that she too will contract the disease. In the face of it all, she decided to stay and thankfully celebrate the gift of life that Tom had each day.

In addition, Tom and Ruth had wonderfully strong support from their church. It would have been so easy for this church to adopt the response of the elder brother in that parable. Rather, the church chose to struggle with demonstrating the response of the father. At one point, Tom said that he had no words to express what he felt about what the response of the church meant to him. More specifically, he said, "I am convinced that one of the reasons I am alive today is because of the strength and encouragement that the people from the church have given. I could have given in long ago, but they have helped me hang in there." Regular calls from church people each week made all the difference in the world for him.

There is real power in recognizing the responsiveness that is a part of us from creation. Our response as the church to those with AIDS will be greatly strengthened by our coming to terms with this part of our theology. Struggling with our theology of creation is essential. Dealing with the questions of what God made when we were created and what God intends for us to do and be are crucial to the church's responding in a healthy and redemptive manner to those who are living with AIDS.

4

A Ministry to All People

Not only is what we believe about God important for our ministry; what we also believe about the role and purpose of Jesus Christ will affect our response to persons with AIDS. In a sense, Jesus' ministry is a model for us. Everything Christ did pointed or aimed people to God. For him, the act of ministry, not the circumstances of the person or place, was of paramount importance. Jesus focused on the need of the person because that was the surest way to make clear what he was about. He sought to reflect the One whom he represented. There are numerous places, especially in John's Gospel (John 1:14; 7:18; 8:50; 11:40; 17:22–23), where Jesus openly indicated that the reason for his presence and his ministry was to glorify and honor his Father.

As we review the events of the ministry of Jesus, four characteristics become evident: inclusiveness, consistency, judgment, and touch.

Inclusiveness

For Christ to have focused on the circumstances of ministry would have revealed an inconsistency and partiality in the nature of God that simply does not exist. There were loaded social issues in Jesus' day, as there are in ours. There were those people whose situations were less socially acceptable than others, such as the Samaritan woman at the well, lepers, and adulterous women. Then there were people who were not acceptable to the religious establishment of Jesus' day, such as Zacchaeus, Matthew, and those called "publicans and sinners." The kind of ministry recorded by the Gospels is a ministry that reveals a strong personal move toward people, with the message that all people and all circumstances are acceptable in God's presence. The inclusiveness of Jesus' ministry brought its own strong, clear honoring of the person of God.

This very inclusiveness stands before the church as an example as we deal with our response to life. Within that example are several significant facts that need to be considered. First of all is the unquestionable fact that Jesus' example declares that all people are acceptable to God. Further, they are acceptable as they are, regardless of their circumstances or condition.

It is important to reread that passage from Luke's Gospel (4:16–20) that has been called the "inaugural address" of Jesus. Jesus had come back to his home church. He was invited to read from the scripture there in the synagogue. Jesus used this opportunity to declare boldly not only who he was as the Anointed One but also, specifically, what he was going to be about. In essence, Jesus was saying that in order to understand who the Messiah is and therefore who God is, pay close attention to the kinds of people that are the recipients of ministry. He chose that wonderful and moving passage from Isaiah 61:

> The Spirit of the Lord GOD is upon me;
>   because the LORD has anointed me
> to bring good tidings to the afflicted;
>   he has sent me to bind up the brokenhearted,
> to proclaim liberty to the captives,
>   and the opening of the prison to those who are bound;
> to proclaim the year of the LORD's favor.

I am never with people with AIDS that these words do not ring in my mind. Whether they are innocent victims or victims of their own behavior, they are nonetheless afflicted each day with this disease and bound by all its effects: physical, social, emotional, and spiritual. The ministry of the church simply must reflect the kind of acceptance, the kind of sensitivity, the kind of relationship that will result in their finally being free, not just physically in death but also free because they have made peace—with themselves, with their God, and with their families and friends. Herein lies the essence of true ministry. For the church to respond to that in the strong example of Jesus Christ is indeed our challenge.

Jesus seemed to go out of his way to be involved with persons whom the religious community had either put in their place (i.e., beggars, women, Samaritans, publicans, and tax collectors) or discarded (i.e., lepers, the handicapped, the emotionally and mentally ill). There was bound to have been plenty of need within the more "acceptable" community for Jesus to have ministered there. However, he chose dramatically to go upstream against the norms of society to make the point that *all* people are acceptable. There are no "throwaway people" in the economy of God.

In addition, a careful study of the situations Jesus encountered will reveal that his ministry was an honest response to need. There were no preconditioned statements of belief required before ministry would happen. Jesus is pictured as always moving toward persons and their needs. Sometimes Jesus sought them out; other times, they sought Jesus because of his reputation for responding. Whatever the context, Jesus seemed always willing to move toward human need, without discrimination or condition.

Certainly there were instances where actions were required for healing to be complete (for example: washing in the pool, John 9, or picking up one's bed in order to walk, John 5). However, it was not the pattern of Jesus' ministry to require a statement of faith or commitment to life before he would engage in ministry. There are numerous incidents where the requirements of discipleship are made abundantly clear. These, however, stand apart from the incidents of ministry to human need. Jesus seemed to delight in offering himself and his powers to those in need, regardless of their circumstances or position in life.

When AIDS comes to church, it will most likely come as an uninvited guest. Most of us will have to respond to AIDS after we discover its presence among us. Few of us will go looking for those with AIDS. The important thing is not how AIDS comes to church. It is in being able to respond consistently in the model of Jesus to all those with AIDS who do come.

The ministering acts of Jesus stand on their own worth. All of them point to and honor God. None of them require anything in return. There are, throughout the Gospels, numerous occasions where the process of discipleship was begun as a result of an encounter with Jesus (i.e., Mark 2:1–5). There are other instances where it was faith itself that brought people to an encounter with Jesus (Matt. 9:27–31). There are even those times when forgiveness of sin was expressed by Jesus to someone with no prior discussion of faith or discipleship, and we know nothing of what happened as a result (John 8:1–11). All of which is to say again that human need and situation are, in the model of Jesus, the things that attracted him to people. He constantly seemed to be going out of his way to go through the Samarias of his day, rather than taking the more acceptable route around them.

For some persons with AIDS, considerations of discipleship and faith will most surely be a part of their journey. For others, perhaps not. In either case, there is the singular presence of need that calls us to respond. In neither case do considerations of faith become a requirement in order for the church to respond. We already seem to understand this with our present ministries to groups such as the mentally or physically handicapped, aged, divorced, ill, and infirm. We simply need to include those with AIDS in the same manner.

Consistency

This raises a second matter that comes out of the ministry of Jesus, the issue of consistency. We have become so conditioned by society that, unfortunately, we choose to avoid some issues. Sticky issues for society are also sticky issues for the church. At the top of that list of issues are things sexual. The church is guilty of treating these kinds of issues unlike the way we treat others.

As an example, let us assume we agree on the theological statement that our bodies are the temple of God. The way we treat our bodies and the things we do with them should reflect an understanding of that biblical truth. For example, there is a minister who abuses his body through overeating and lack of exercise and becomes grossly overweight. Then there is another minister who takes his body into a series of adulterous relationships. When disclosure happens, chances are that only one of them will lose his job, and it will not be the one who eats too well.

Another example: There are two church members. One of them exposes his body to enough alcohol and tobacco that cancer develops and death occurs. The other exposes his body to enough promiscuous sexual activity that AIDS is contracted and death occurs. Chances are that we will not hesitate to support the one who dies from cancer. To the one with AIDS, we will usually be very cautious indeed about being involved.

Another example needs to be drawn. Because the majority of AIDS cases are related to the homosexual issue, there is often a great deal of resistance to being open to them because homosexuality is considered to be so "unnatural." Yet little is said about other "unnatural" acts, such as parents abusing children or spouses abusing each other physically and sexually. In addition, there are the deeply damaging effects of emotional abuse that we inflict on each other as adult-to-adult and parent-to-child. Nowhere in God's plan for us can these acts be called natural.

We are woefully inconsistent in our response to people and situations. Yet the biblical record is clearly consistent. A careful examination of scripture will reveal that sins are not graded or scaled. Contextually, they are generally treated together, with none singled out as worse than the others.

Jesus sought to minister from a perspective of consistency in a society that surely graded things and scaled them as "better than" or "worse than." He wanted to make clear that it is the person involved in a situation who is important. Situations and circumstances should never preclude ministry. Consistency is one way to assure that they do not.

The Bible treats references to homosexuality in the context of other issues that people struggle with in life. Paul's letter to the Corinthians (1 Cor. 6:9–10, KJV) is often quoted regarding homosexuality. What is not often noted or quoted is that Paul names a whole list of "unrighteous" things, including fornication, idolatry, adultery, homosexuality. thievery, drunkenness, slandering, and swindling. Our lack of consistency enables us to treat sexually related problems like AIDS quite differently from things that are nonsexual and thus more socially acceptable. The person who cheats on income tax and the person who passes along slanderous gossip about others are in the same category, biblically, as those who are involved in sexual matters such as fornication, adultery, or homosexuality. In God's summary statement of an ethical and moral basis for living, called the Decalogue, or the Ten Commandments, only one reference is made to sexual matters, and that is to adultery, not homosexuality or promiscuity.

The Old Testament is as consistent as the New Testament. The passage is often quoted from Leviticus regarding homosexuality (18:22). Yet rarely are similar references cited to those parts of Leviticus that talk about stoning to death those caught in adultery or stoning to death those sons who become unmanageable in their behavior, as is outlined in Deuteronomy 21. I am not suggesting that we become less concerned with any issue. I am suggesting that we become consistent in our concern and not let our preoccupation prevent us from ministering in the model of Jesus.

We have already moved in the area of AIDS to grading from more acceptable to unacceptable those who contract the disease. While I had thought of some AIDS patients as "innocent victims," I had not really ranked them in order of acceptability. Larry's mother mentioned it in a conversation after his death. Her comment was that, as far as the church is concerned with people with AIDS, the list would run like this, from most acceptable to unacceptable: (1) infants born with AIDS; (2) persons who were infected from blood transfusions; (3) spouses of persons with AIDS who contracted it before they knew the other had it; (4) those contracting the disease from promiscuity; and (5) those contracting the disease from adultery. Then she paused and said, "It would probably be a toss-up as to who would be on the bottom of the list, the prostitutes, the addicts, or the gays." There is an unfortunate amount of truth in her assessment.

Judgment

A third matter that needs to be lifted up and examined is the issue of judgment. Jesus was clear, beyond any question, that judging is not our task or our business, but God's. In fact, Jesus reminds us not only that we will be judged but also that our judgments of others will be judged as well. In regard to AIDS, our judgment of others often comes from an emotional frame of reference rather than a theological one. What we do not understand or like or even admit the possibility of in ourselves is usually that on which we pass the harshest judgment. Whatever our frame of reference, there is a theological dimension to the issue of accountability.

The essence of the gospel is "good news." Many people who are living with AIDS hardly ever hear *any* good news. What they hear first and loudest is the message that they are in big trouble with this world and with God because of their behavior or their lifestyle. This pronouncement of the bad news of judgment, punishment, and wrath, in the name of One who represents all things good, is a self-contradictory message. Judgmental bad news can be communicated non-verbally as well. We can just withdraw from those with AIDS. We can refuse to touch them or speak to them or look at them or include them. Judgment can be expressed both ways. Neither way is theologically consistent with the persons and work of Jesus.

Some feel that a posture of judgment is necessary in order to call for repentance and a change of lifestyle from people. To capitalize on someone's tragic circumstances for the purpose of evangelism falls far short of the example of Jesus given throughout the Gospels. Such an approach is reminiscent of long-ago days when slaves were transported from Africa to the new country of America. It was not at all uncommon in those days to stop en route to evangelize the slaves, on the theory, perhaps, that Christian slaves would bring a more handsome profit in the marketplace. The slaves received two messages. One message was, As white people we will shun you and avoid you and not accept you as people. The second message was, While we have you in shackles, we want you to know that Jesus loves you and we are brothers and sisters. Such double messages not only end in hopeless confusion but make a mockery of the example and ministry of Christ.

The attempt to relate judgmentally to persons with AIDS is much like that. We send two messages to them as well. One is, We will shun you, avoid you, not touch you, and not accept you as fully human; you are a second-class citizen at best. The second message is, While you are shackled in the death trap called AIDS, we want you to know that Jesus loves you and we really are brothers and sisters.

A very acute description of judgment, one which should be emblazoned on our minds and hearts as we minister to persons with AIDS, comes from Frederick Buechner in his delightful little book of theological definitions, *Wishful Thinking*. In reminding us that judgment waits in the future for all of us, Buechner emphasizes that judgments about us and our lives will take place, but judgment will also happen on our judgments of others. Not only will we be judged by God, who is the ultimate judge, but we will also be judged by Christ, who is the one who loves us more than any other.[7]

We may need to do some rethinking about evangelism in light of the situation of AIDS patients. The proclamation of the good news and the invitation for everyone to make the kind of commitment that results in discipleship are essential parts of the evangelical church tradition. However, there are many situations where any kind of ministry can be subverted by conditional calls for repentance and renunciation of lifestyles and habits.

One of the saddest examples of this was reported by Larry's mother. During one of Larry's stays in the hospital, his mother had the opportunity to meet another mother whose son was also dying of AIDS. With great pain, Larry's mother told me of this other woman's daily trips to the hospital, where she sat by her son's bed, reminding him that unless he repented and renounced his lifestyle, he would surely burn in hell for all eternity. It was not until just a couple of days before his death that she realized this approach was not only nonproductive, it was separating her from her son for what precious time they had left.

As a pastor, I have a deep conviction about and concern for every person's relationship with God, especially those whose life is drawing to a close. However, rather than condemning and judging and calling for repentance, I have found that I just need to be present to the religious issues that are already surfacing. The presence of God helps me to be sensitive to what is already beginning to happen in the lives of people dying with AIDS. If I contain myself long enough, there is ample opportunity to discuss with any AIDS patient what is involved in getting one's life ready for death. In my experience, without exception, one of the major issues that those dying with AIDS face is the need to have assurance that the sins of their lives, whatever their nature, are forgiven. Moments of such confession in the context of pastoral care are sacred moments for anyone.

As the disease of AIDS progresses, the issue of renunciation of lifestyles and habits becomes a moot point. Whether the lifestyle through which AIDS was contracted was sexual or drug-related, the disease itself puts an end to further activity in either area. To impose such concerns upon someone who is approaching death is to miss the point of what is happening. Whatever our concern about a person's relationship with God, a sensitive pastoral presence will provide more than enough opportunity to deal with any aspect of this issue.

Touch

A final matter needs to be lifted out for examination as we look at the life and ministry of Jesus as our model and example. That is the importance of touch, the laying on of hands. Until one has walked awhile in the darkness with persons with AIDS, one cannot begin to imagine how very significant touch is. The initial reaction to AIDS is often not well thought out. It has been called AIDS hysteria. Some journals have named it, more specifically, AFRAIDS (Acute Fear Regarding AIDS).[8] Whatever it is called, the result is loss of contact in general and touch in particular by the AIDS patient. The reaction has been painfully witnessed in those situations where children have contracted AIDS through blood transfusions. Enormous battles have erupted in communities and on school boards as to whether these children should attend school with other children. It is difficult to imagine any human being having to do without touch. To be a child and to lose that kind of interaction with other human beings is truly devastating.

We have made of AIDS a kind of modern-day leprosy and, of AIDS patients themselves, modern-day lepers. They have become the untouchables in our society. Medical data assure us that there is no risk in touching a person who has AIDS. However, there is also a biblical rationale for this

all-important ministry of touch. Recall the numerous instances where healing was associated with the laying on of
Jesus' hands. While touching is not the same as healing,
there is a kind of healing that goes with being touched by
people who care about you and care for you. It is so comforting to be touched in times of crisis. Many times during
a death experience, I have simply held on to someone in a
desperate kind of hug, because there were no words to say.
Touching another in the name of Jesus Christ is a kind of
healing all by itself.

In the eighth chapter of Matthew (vs. 1–3), an encounter
between Jesus and a leper is recorded. The leper approached Jesus asking for healing. Jesus stretched forth his
hand and touched the leper, and he was healed. The gospel
writer used the word "touch" to dramatize how different
this act of Jesus was. He could just as easily have said that
Jesus healed the man. The writer was making a point that
not even lepers were off limits to Jesus: "He stretched out
his hand and touched him." As far as society was concerned,
healing was one thing, but touching an untouchable was
something else entirely.

Tom shared with me an experience he had with touching.
As his illness progressed, his participation and attendance
in church understandably declined. Word began to get
around that Tom indeed had AIDS. After he had been ab-
sent from church for several Sundays, he came one Sunday
morning and took his usual seat alongside Ruth, down front
on the east side of the sanctuary. I was not aware that
anything special happened that day. I remember that I
along with others was really glad to see Tom well enough
to be in church again. But later Tom told me that the neat-
est thing about being back was that, even though everyone
knew he had AIDS, people still touched him on Sunday
morning.

He had come to church fully expecting to be shunned.
Surely, he felt, those who normally shook his hand or
hugged him would not do so now. However, he went on, the
special thing was that Estelle came down to where he was

seated and made him stand up so she could hug him. The best part was that she waited until almost eleven o'clock, when the church was full of people, before she walked down front to his seat, knowing that everybody in the church could see her not only touch him but hug him.

Estelle is our treasurer, and one of the very favorite special people around this church. Everybody loves and kids with her and enjoys being around her. Her quiet ministry of touch did not go unnoticed, either by Tom or by a host of others.

Whatever else happened in worship that day, for Tom the Word had already become flesh in that act of touching. In that simple, bold, strong act of a fellow church member, Tom felt the good news of Jesus Christ. He heard through the gift of touch the words of the father in Luke's story (15:11–32), You are loved, you are prized, and you are welcomed home.

5

Ministering to Families of Persons with AIDS

In looking back over almost three years of ministry to persons with AIDS, especially those related to our congregation, I am struck by the amount of time and energy that has been spent with family members. Of course, any time there is pastoral involvement in a terminal illness, there will almost always be interaction with the family. However, with AIDS there are complexities that merit particular attention. Let me share some general principles that apply to all family members and then be specific in terms of ministry related to the parents, the children, and the spouses of those with AIDS.

Information and Support

One of the first things families will need is basic information about the disease itself. Regardless of how well read people may be, the presence of a crisis often calls for the reintroduction of information. My own understanding of AIDS was greatly augmented when Tom and Ruth invited me to share in their process of education by going with them to doctors and support groups. Over the years, we constantly exchanged information.

There are many questions families usually have that are crucial to their understanding. When the family is trying to process all the implications of the disease, these questions will run the gamut from death to personal hygiene. People in the medical community are not always able to take the time to go into the kind of detail that is needed. In addition, they often do not have the kind of relationship to the family that a pastor has.

When the AIDS patient is at home, family members will have questions about such matters as personal hygiene or special needs in relation to housekeeping, because of concern about possible infection. A woman whose husband had AIDS experienced a great deal of pressure from both her husband and his family to "clean out the house" to be sure no one else caught the disease. "Cleaning out the house" meant, to them, burning all sheets, blankets, and mattresses; sterilizing all pots, pans, silverware, and dishes; and having the whole house fumigated. While this seemed a bit much to her, she nonetheless was not sure what was needed. Basic information took care of her concerns.

The pastor does not need to become the resident expert on AIDS. But one of the most needed services is the provision of reliable information. Such information can be obtained from local sources such as the American Red Cross, local public health offices and AIDS centers, and national public health offices. A list of addresses is included in the appendix of this book. The single best resource piece to place in a family's hands is the *Surgeon General's Report on Acquired Immune Deficiency Syndrome.* It is clear, easy to understand, and speaks to the very points that families are raising.

Knowing what one is up against in a time of crisis is the first step toward being able to deal effectively with what will come. When AIDS appears in the context of pastoral relationships, the stage is set for providing a family with needed information. Trust and openness between the family and the pastor make the situation really excellent for helping families prepare for the road that lies ahead. Even in those situations where the family and the pastor do not have much if any relationship, it is not uncommon for the same kind of openness toward a minister to be present. The minister enjoys the unique privilege of having an open door in most times of crisis, regardless of the depth of the relationship.

A second thing that families related to AIDS seem to need is an immense amount of reassurance. This need seems to focus around several very specific issues. First and foremost, once again, is the issue of confidentiality. There is a great deal of concern about who will find out about AIDS being in their family and what effect that knowledge will have. Most families know at least one horror story related to AIDS. Most of these stories involve the way in which the families themselves experienced rejection or abuse. Wives, especially, seem to be concerned, if they are employed, that their own workplaces not be affected by information about the presence of AIDS in their homes. Ruth said on more than one occasion how important it was to have a neutral place like work where she did not have to confront what she did elsewhere in her life.

The issue of confidentiality is sometimes as important to the family members as to the person with AIDS. Even though the legal situation is improving in regard to the forced termination of employment of persons with AIDS, families continue to be concerned about confidentiality. A part of this response has to do with their own fears that if people around them know, perhaps they, too, will be rejected. For families to watch someone they love struggle with fears about isolation and rejection while they are moving toward death is difficult enough. To have to deal with those same fears themselves makes the whole dynamic difficult to manage.

This issue is often brought into focus around the question of where to have the funeral service when a person with AIDS dies. In situations where the church and the minister have the opportunity to relate to both the AIDS patient and the family, there can be some real issues, especially when the AIDS patient is a homosexual. More often than not, the families of those persons have continued participating in their own church. Their church community may not know, for instance, that there is a homosexual family member who is dying with AIDS. In many cases where disclosure has happened, as in Larry's situation, the original church has judgmentally withdrawn fellowship or sent subtle messages that "folks like that" are not welcome.

Often, the parents of children who are active in a gay church do not themselves feel comfortable enough to have the funeral service there. They may also want to keep the sexual identity and illness a matter of private knowledge and thus prefer to have the service in a traditional church. As with Larry's funeral, the ministers of the gay church in our community are very understanding and supportive of such situations.

Hence the choice of the place of the funeral service becomes a very complex and important issue. It is crucial that pastors remain sensitive to this dynamic. In addition, ministers need to be very generous in offering their buildings for such funerals. If the situation includes people who are not involved or are away from their own church community, the offer of local church buildings can be extremely important and helpful. For many, the church building can become a neutral place where the important ritual of the funeral service can take place and also meet the needs of the family at that time in terms of their own fears of disclosure.

I held the service of an AIDS patient in our church when neither the young man nor his parents were members. They had gone through the very difficult time of being rejected by their own church in another community as a result of disclosure about the presence of homosexuality in their family. As a result, church had been abandoned for almost ten years, although their son had become very active in the gay church in his community. The family did not want to have the funeral service at the gay church. Our building offered them a way to move through a very difficult time in their lives with the security of tradition. As a friend pointed out, some months later, we had in a very quiet way become a contemporary version of the Old Testament "city of refuge" for this family. The physical place of the funeral had become a significant expression of biblical truth. Having the service here gave this family the gift of being able to deal with their needs in a place of security and safety. Our church became a place where human interaction and community could happen without any fear of disclosure of any detail regarding the lifestyle or death of this family member. It was a place of biblical refuge in a time of real need.

Families also need assurance that their pastor is going to stick by them. Early on, AIDS families have no real idea of what is ahead. There is simply the overwhelming presence of tragedy and the disruption of life for them all. Whatever lies ahead is bearable if they do not have to go through it alone. Here the pastor or ministering person needs to count the cost prior to involvement. That is why the earlier chapters of this book unfold as they do. It would be better not to get involved at all with a family who is dealing with AIDS, than to get involved and then for some reason abandon them in midstream.

From a biblical perspective, the words of Jesus are quite plain as they relate to discipleship. In the Gospel of Luke, Jesus tells the story of counting the cost as it relates to following him in service and ministry (Luke 14:25–35). Ministry comes as an outgrowth of discipleship. Dealing with families with AIDS is a contemporary expression of this dynamic in terms of the church and its ministers being able to give families all possible assurance that they will not be abandoned in the middle of the process.

This kind of assurance takes on critical dimensions when the possibility of suicide arises. It is not uncommon for anyone with a terminal illness to contemplate suicide. Because of the often long-drawn-out process of dying, coupled with social and emotional isolation, suicide is a very common consideration among those suffering with AIDS.

Interestingly enough, both wives in our congregation with husbands dying with AIDS had to deal with this issue. Central to all the feelings of fear and anger that go with such consideration is the need to be assured that their pastor and church will not desert them if their husbands do commit suicide. Coming home from work each day to confront the presence of AIDS in the family is a heavy enough load for any wife. To have to consider the possibility of coming home to find that death has been hastened by suicide really complicates things.

Because suicide is always a possibility, it is extremely important that families feel assured that their minister will stay with them all the way.

Families also should feel that their needs will not be ignored or forgotten. It is so easy for the minister to focus on the one dying. So many things are happening all at once both with the patient and with the person ministering that it is easy to overlook the family. It is extremely important to find ways to be in touch with family members outside of the setting where the AIDS patient is. My visits to see Tom and Ruth at their home were important. However, even with Ruth present, the visit focused on Tom. Therefore, I tried consistently to call Ruth at work, with her permission, just to tell her that she and what she was dealing with were important to me.

This need becomes especially crucial for children whose parents are dying with AIDS. They are often easier to overlook than the spouse. It is vital to spend time dealing with their concerns. Many times the only way to do that is to make time to spend alone with the child in order to focus on his or her questions or concerns.

A third general area of importance is the need to reaffirm that we are dealing with the normal grief process as a part of the journey of AIDS. While this perspective will no doubt come naturally for those with some years of ministering experience, it is sufficiently important that everyone needs to be reminded of it.

We can get so caught up in all the unique complexities of ministering to persons with AIDS we may forget that many things in this process are quite normal. Certain reactions are experienced by all people dealing with terminal illness. In talking with Larry's parents after his death, I asked them to share with me some things that they found as parents of an AIDS patient that were especially helpful to them during Larry's illness. Immediately, they said that they needed all the things that were just a part of the normal grief process. They were saying, "Don't forget that there is a side of this disease that is as normal as any other kind of terminal illness."

It will be helpful for those who are ministering to persons with AIDS to review the grief process and the steps that most people experience. This review will enable those who are providing ministry to keep things in balance and not overlook some of the really significant issues.

In addition to these general concerns, there are items that relate to specific family members. Parents, spouses, and children of persons with AIDS all have their own unique agendas to deal with. Being sensitive to them can be immensely helpful as they go through this process.

Parents of AIDS Patients

Parents with grown sons or daughters who are dying with AIDS will generally fall into one of two groups. The first is those who are in the same location with their child. Often that child has come home because there is no other place to go. The second is those parents who are living in one place while the child who is suffering with AIDS is living somewhere else.

For parents whose children have AIDS, one of the first questions they may need to face is whether or not that child can come home once the disease has been diagnosed. For some parents this will not be an issue at all. Their child is ill and needs to be cared for, and their home is open. For others, it is a bit more complex, especially in those situations where an adult child has been gone from home for some time and has not maintained close contact. Many times, children who are gay or heavily into the drug scene have consciously distanced themselves from their parents, to protect the parents from having to deal with a lifestyle with which they might not agree, or to protect the child from having to deal with the hassle of possible rejection by the parents. It is not uncommon for children to leave home and assume lifestyles that are simply never disclosed to their parents.

Parents who are dealing with this, whatever shape it takes, will certainly need someone with whom they can discuss their feelings. The pastoral relationship provides an excellent setting. However, good pastoral care can happen only if there is sensitivity to the possibility of some or even all of these dynamics going on in people's lives.

Parents who are living somewhere other than where their ill children are pose yet another set of circumstances. It is important to understand what impact geographical distance has on their relationship before trying to deal with the issue of the presence of AIDS. If the situation is like that of most dispersed families, a number of things affect the relationship. There will probably be more parents living in this kind of situation than those who live near their children with AIDS. A supportive relationship from their minister and the church seems crucial in providing a safe place where what the parents feel can be dealt with. Often, guilt and anger will surface. Unfortunately, these folks are often left alone to deal with these feelings. A supportive relationship with a minister would seem to be vital to those dealing with AIDS at a distance. One of the most practical things that can be done is for a contact to be made with a sensitive minister near where the distant patient or parents reside. This can be a strong and beautiful way to bridge the gap in relationships created by distance.

There are, however, two words of caution. Any such contact with a distant minister about the presence of AIDS in a family needs to be made only after permissions have been given by all parties involved. If an AIDS patient would like the family to have the support of a minister, it is crucial to be sure that the family involved wants a minister to know. When the family lives at some distance from the AIDS patient, it is very easy for them to want no one else around them to know what is happening.

A young AIDS patient in Miami was concerned that his grandmother did not have any support to carry her through this crisis save her own private faith. When I contacted her at his request, she was deeply moved by his concern, but emphatic in not wanting anyone, ministers included, to know what was going on in her extended family. As painful as it was for me to do so, I respected her wishes. I tried to help only by sending occasional notes and cards and calling her on the telephone as she waited for the death of her grandson.

This matter seems a bit easier when concerned parents want some ministering presence for a child who has AIDS. While there may be resistance to the presence of a "professional religious person" on the part of some AIDS patients, most seem open to the expression of care and concern. In the face of the reality of death, the religious dimension of life becomes more apparent. Since most AIDS patients are treated in fairly large medical facilities, most of them will have some kind of chaplain service available. Calling the chaplain can be a way to initiate a contact.

A second word of caution is that one must be extremely careful as to the theological and emotional posture of the person to whom the referral is made. With the wide variety of reactions from the religious community in response to AIDS, one cannot be too careful in this area of referrals. It would almost be better for a patient or family to face AIDS alone than to have to endure the presence of an insensitive, judgmental, or overzealous minister. If checking and re-checking results in healthy, religious support being available to those dealing with AIDS, it is well worth the effort.

In many instances, the minister stands as one of the few persons, if not the only one, to whom families in this situation can turn during this time. Confidentiality is always a very real issue, and if the parents and the person with AIDS do not live in the same area, this is especially true. The need for the person with AIDS to come back home after having been away for a long while can pose a problem. Families may have been going about their own lives very quietly while their child lived elsewhere. The thought of reabsorbing an adult child back into the home can be traumatic in itself. To do so in the presence of AIDS is much more difficult.

Regular pastoral contacts are essential because they provide an outlet to discuss what is really going on in the lives of AIDS patients. To be able sensitively to help families deal with the reality of what is and the impending reality of what is coming is a pastoral and ministering gift in the best sense of the word.

Support groups for parents of adult children with AIDS provide an excellent context for families to work these problems out with others who are dealing with essentially the same issues. Many larger metropolitan communities have such groups already established. Where no groups exist, a church could help in organizing one. Perhaps all that is needed is the offer of a meeting place. Perhaps there is a need for leadership, which can come from within the congregation. Pastors and churches need to be aware of these specific ways they can be of help.

In those communities where only two or three families in a given church are touched by AIDS, it is still important that mutual support be given. Perhaps the pastor can be the one who gently and compassionately brings the families together. It would be helpful for ministers to pay close attention to what is happening in other churches in order to explore the possibility of linking together families from various churches for their mutual support. Of course, such contacts are made only with the express permission of the families involved. The issue of confidentiality cannot be stressed too strongly.

I found it particularly moving to introduce to each other the two wives in our congregation whose husbands were dying with AIDS. Because of Tom and Ruth's openness about AIDS, Ruth was known to Elaine, but even though Ruth and Tom knew there was another family touched with AIDS in our congregation, they did not know who it was. In talking with Elaine, it became apparent to me that she indeed wanted to talk to Ruth but hesitated to go to her on her own. I secured permission from both of them, and they began in their own quiet way to share with each other. However much information and help the medical community and the religious community provide, it pales in comparison to what one wife can tell another wife about living with the reality that your husband is dying with AIDS. Linking such women together in their common need is one of the strongest kinds of ministry a pastor can provide.

Children of AIDS Patients

Children of families touched with AIDS present yet another dynamic. Here in Plantation, children of both families are in their teens or early twenties. It is interesting that even though one family found out about AIDS almost two years after the other, the reaction and response of the children was practically identical.

One of the most prominent issues to be dealt with in children is the fear of losing the other parent. In both families, the children were concerned and preoccupied with the possibility that they would lose their mother as well. The dynamic of fear is naturally laced with the strong thread of anger. Children who have an understanding of how AIDS is contracted have a heightened sense of fear, rooted in anger. To lose a parent or stepparent is bad enough. To face the possibility of becoming orphaned is almost overwhelming to a child or young person. To have that death come about because of AIDS makes anger very understandable and real.

Ruth's daughter is in her early twenties. With all that was already going on in her life, the threat of losing her mother as well was almost more than she could stand. Through her tears she cried out, "If my mother gets AIDS and dies because of him, all I have to say is that he had better die first!" And then she topped off her anger with this statement of real fear: "Because then I will not have anybody. I will be all alone." I wanted to reach across the room and gather her in my arms as you would a small child who is suddenly very frightened.

Elaine's children were preoccupied with the same agenda, though not quite as intensely; they were just beginning their journey. Nonetheless, the fear and potential anger were there, ready to burst forth.

Because of the apparent good health of both Ruth and Elaine, it was a temptation to assure their children that things were going to be all right, and they really did not need to worry. In both situations I pointed out that having healthy mothers was certainly in their favor at this point, and they did not need to let their fears rob them of whatever good days were present right now. I assured them that I had talked with their mothers about taking the blood test for the presence of the virus. Since taking this test was a decision each mother would have to make, I encouraged them to discuss the issue. I assured them their mothers could handle talking about this, and they did not need to be afraid of raising the question.

I reminded them of the words of reassurance found in the King James Version of the Twenty-third Psalm, especially verse 4, "Yea, though I walk through the valley of the shadow of death, I will fear no evil: for thou art with me; thy rod and thy staff they comfort me." God does not promise us a way around that valley. When crises come, there is only one way, and that is straight through. Even though they may not understand why they have to take that route, and even though it may seem unfair, there is a note of good news: they do not have to do it alone. They do not need to fear, for the promise and the presence of God will go with them.

I also related the "no fear" phrase to the good news of the gospel of Jesus Christ, reminding them that the first words of proclamation about the birth of Christ were the words of the angels, "Fear not." But no matter how assuring such biblical words may be, these young people still had to make their own journey through the "valley of AIDS."

Often, the very discussion of death with adolescents calls forth an immense amount of projection and transference. They begin to wonder whether they too will die from this disease. Providing them with basic information about AIDS and how it is contracted is essential. The Surgeon General's report is the best single piece of literature that can be given to them, too. It is factual and direct, and easy for most adolescents to read and understand.

In regard to the children of AIDS patients, there is another area of concern that has not yet surfaced. While I was working in the field of institutional child care, I became acutely aware of the large number of young teenage girls who have been victims of incest. As AIDS spreads into the heterosexual community, there will inevitably be teenage girls who have been sexually assaulted by fathers or other men in their families who may have been exposed to AIDS. The young girls are going to have to deal with the fear that they too might get AIDS. Sexual assault and incest are in themselves very difficult issues for teenage girls to handle. Many teenagers already know that AIDS is basically a sexually transmitted disease, so we are bound to have many such young women also having to deal with yet another real fear.

Spouses of AIDS Patients

The spouses of those with AIDS present yet another unique opportunity. From the start, they are the persons who must maintain stability for the family once the presence of AIDS is disclosed. As the disease spreads in the heterosexual community in the future, more and more spouses, most of them wives, will have to carry this burden. They will be emotionally and relationally involved as well as legally responsible for making many decisions as the illness progresses. A sensitive pastor can be of real aid in helping spouses sort out their roles and providing them with resources to accomplish those tasks.

Uppermost in the minds of many spouses, just after concern for their own health and the issue of confidentiality, is worry about money. Even families with good insurance can be devastated by medical bills. The problem becomes even greater, of course, when the person with AIDS is unable to continue working.

I was able to direct Tom and Ruth to an attorney in our congregation who helped Ruth to know what was ahead financially and what she could or should be doing. With his advice, they were able to begin to deal with financial realities one step at a time.

The need of the spouse to have ongoing emotional support cannot be stressed too strongly. On a day-to-day basis, the role of stabilizer of the family is a giant task. To become overly consumed with AIDS is to give the disease more power than it should have. Many normal things continue each day, not only because they need to get done but also because of the symbol they provide that life is indeed bigger than AIDS. Such simple tasks as grocery shopping, grass cutting, and housecleaning are important. The pastor needs to affirm the place of these things as families cope with AIDS. Perhaps other persons can help in bearing the load of daily living. This is especially true when there are children still at home. Normal everyday things that continue to happen as they always have provide great, silent assurance to children and young people that life still goes on.

Early one Sunday afternoon, Tom called me to express his worry that Ruth was going down the tubes with the load she was carrying. I dropped by the house. It was obvious from one look at Ruth that she was about stressed out. Not knowing what else to do and not having anything specific to offer, I asked what could we do to help her. With great emotion, she began to talk about her need to have some people to talk to who knew what was going on. (We were still at that stage where confidentiality was important because of Tom's job.) While she had plenty of people around her with whom she could do normal kinds of things, they did not—and, in her mind, could not—know that Tom was dying with AIDS. Confidentiality, as important as it was, became a source of real conflict within her. She found herself constantly thinking, when around friends and neighbors, that if they really knew what was going on with her husband at home, they would not want to be around her at all.

As I grasped the enormity of her heartbreak, I realized that there was indeed something we at church could do for her. Because it seemed so important for some people to know what was going on in Ruth's world, I asked her to give me the names of several women at church with whom she could feel comfortable. With her permission, I would invite them to become part of a very quiet support system.

She gave me the names of five women whom she and Tom agreed I could contact. I called them one by one on the phone and asked them to come to my office for a meeting after services that Sunday evening. I did not go into detail on the phone but stressed the importance of what I needed to talk with them about. Each of them agreed, no questions asked, although I did sense that curiosity was running high.

As soon as the service was over, I met them in my office and carefully and gently disclosed what Tom and Ruth were dealing with. I told them what Ruth needed and how I felt they could be of help. I outlined three things very clearly. First, they needed to go home and talk with their families and secure their blessing. (Tom and Ruth had agreed that this was important, even though there was some risk involved.) Second, I stressed how important confidentiality was at this point. It was of paramount importance that no one else in the church besides them and their families know all the facts. Later, when Tom was unable to work and confidentiality became less of an issue, they could then relax in this area. Third, I stressed that they needed to be prepared to go with Ruth for the duration. This was no four- or six-week assignment. They would have to be willing to be present with Ruth "from this day forward."

By the providence of God, our deacons were meeting in the next room with a guest, a very good friend from Hospice Care, who was doing some training with them in ministry to those with terminal illness. Polly and her staff had already been involved with AIDS patients. As soon as she was through, I asked her to spend a few minutes with these women, telling them specifically about the medical aspects of AIDS. I knew she could say things this group of women needed to hear in a way I could not. I felt the presence of God in that room. An incredible thing was happening. In a significant way, Ruth was about to experience the Word becoming flesh for her. In an equally significant way, this group of women were about to discover ministry in ways they had never known before.

After our discussion, the room was very quiet. Then one woman looked up and said perceptively, "Well, pastor, I don't think this is going to be just a ministry of green beans." How very right she was! As important as is the ministry of taking green beans when and where needed, there was no way to measure the importance of the response to the call of God to this ministry.

The women began their task in a beautifully quiet way, as Ruth's own description shows: "The very next day they all had contacted me in their own special way. A couple of them phoned me. One came by with a flower and a card. It was a real relief to finally have someone who knew what was really going on. Each of these ladies had qualities I admired. They were all special to me in their own ways. They have truly been my support system. I have been blessed to have made these special friendships, and they continue to this day."

What Ruth discovered out of her own need was a community of integrity in the strong name of Jesus Christ. Here were several women who were willing to risk involvement in an area that was fairly new to all of us because of their faith relationship with Ruth. Their very presence affirmed normalcy in Ruth's life. They knew all the facts and chose to help. No longer did Ruth have to deal with the fear of possibly being rejected by women friends if they found out about Tom.

Sometimes all of them would meet and go out for a meal. Other times, just one or two of them would get together with Ruth. The form their meetings took was not the issue. What was important and lifegiving to Ruth was the fact that they were willing to "pitch their tent" in her world.

That was in 1985. Even though Ruth's needs are different now, this group still stays in touch. Their schedule is a bit more flexible, but their significance is nonetheless important. Ruth has been the grateful recipient of the grace of God through the quiet ministry of these women.

Remember, this all happened without others in the church ever knowing anything about it. Five women, their husbands, and their children were told about Ruth and Tom in confidence. The fact that confidentiality has basically remained intact is yet another sign of the grace of God. It also says that when ministry focuses on the needs of people, you can trust those whom God calls out to do what needs to be done.

Not until early 1987, in discussing this book with the congregation one Wednesday evening, did the larger church even have any idea that ministry of this significance and magnitude had been happening all around them without their knowing it. In recalling this part of the journey with Tom and Ruth, I am filled with deep humility and gratitude at the privilege of being pastor of this church in general and these people in particular.

As with the children of persons with AIDS, another very special issue will be facing spouses in the future. After the deaths of their husbands, women like Ruth and Elaine will be more than just young widows; they will be "marked widows." As they contemplate the possibility of dating and even marriage in the future, the fact that their husbands died with AIDS will become a real issue in their interpersonal relationships. Given the normal reactions of a cross section of people in society, there is real risk that many men will be immediately turned off at the news of their dates having become widowed through AIDS. It will take an unusual set of circumstances for deepened relationships to develop once this issue is in the open. To disclose is to risk rejection with those with whom relationships seem possible. Yet not to disclose is to run the risk of real problems in the future, not to speak of issues of dishonesty and integrity.

For these two women in our church, and countless others

as time passes, AIDS will not end at the cemetery. It will be part of their lives for as long as they live. Radical new discoveries by the medical community are the only thing that could in any way lessen the load of this particular burden.

Like those five women who were called out to walk with Ruth, the church must be prepared to minister "for the duration." AIDS promises not only to change the nature of our society but to greatly affect the way the church goes about ministry. Becoming aware of some of these difficult issues will be helpful to the church in its response to family members of those dealing with AIDS.

6

Enabling the Church to Respond

The response of a church to AIDS can take many different forms. This chapter suggests various possibilities. While the list is not exhaustive, the ideas given here can be adapted, and they may suggest other ways to aid in the struggle with this issue in your own church community.

Pastoral Care

First of all, good, solid, biblically based pastoral care is vital to ministry to persons and families dealing with AIDS. Good pastoral care begins with a reaffirmation of the need to respond to people with AIDS as persons and not see them primarily in the context of the circumstances in which their disease was contracted. In addition, it is important to remember that the gospel means "good news." Our response to those with AIDS must embody a kind of presence that indeed sounds like good news to them. Being aware of all that these patients may be dealing with is important. There is the initial confrontation with the reality that AIDS is a terminal illness. The pastoral caregiver must appreciate the range of human responses to such news. It is not uncommon to have to deal with feelings of shock, numbness, fear, anger, bargaining with God, fantasy, and denial on the part of anyone dying with a terminal illness.

Creating the awareness of the presence of God by being

present as a pastoral caregiver is the good news setting in which the feelings and dynamics of dying can be processed and responded to by a perceptive person. There is no substitute for a pastoral relationship that can help the person deal with the need for a strengthened faith as he or she moves toward death. Such a relationship can offer support by one's very presence. It can offer a sense of hopefulness to the person that he or she is not being abandoned by God even in the face of this seemingly hopeless situation. A new and deeper understanding of the gift of forgiveness can be a vital part of the pastoral care experience. Such a ministry of being present needs to be strengthened and undergirded with the reading of scripture and prayer together.

In this way pastoral care provides a bold statement of the involvement of God in the person's life. This then opens the way for the emergence of genuine hope and reconciliation for those dealing with AIDS. It also opens the door for other relationships within the patient's own family or circle of friends that need to be faced. The issue of closure in relationships can be crucial to one who is nearing death. The ability to do that with any kind of integrity will come out of a patient's own strengthened faith experience.

The presence of AIDS involves additional complexities to which the pastoral caregiver needs to respond. The impact of AIDS on the body is seen in the breakdown of the immune system, with its subsequent physical problems. The emotional and spiritual impact of AIDS is often seen in the breakdown of one's feelings of self-esteem and personal self-worth. Most often, the central dynamic to be dealt with here is the issue of guilt. It is important for the pastoral caregiver to be able to help the patient sort through all that is related to this issue. This may mean having to listen to some pretty explicit details about past lifestyles and experiences. It is important to do this nonjudgmentally. Listening in love and acceptance of the person wherever he or she is now can be a great gift as the patient processes some of these feelings. Allowing the person to verbalize *all* these feelings, even guilty ones, often provides opportunities to deal with more significant or substantive issues.

Feelings of despair and anxiety often go hand in hand with emotional difficulties related to the issue of self-esteem. The dying person may need an immense amount of emotional and spiritual support. The pastoral caregiver who is competent and comfortable in such situations has an excellent opportunity to follow through on this portion of the journey with AIDS. For those who are not able to do this, referral to someone who *is* comfortable and competent is an equally good gift.

This agenda of deeply felt emotions is additionally compounded by the reaction of others to the person with AIDS. Family and friends may abandon or reject the person when they become aware of the diagnosis. In many instances, the only constant presence that an AIDS patient can count on is that of the pastoral caregiver. The building of a support system from within the church can be an indispensable item in the life of such a patient. This support will assure the person that he or she indeed is not going to be rejected, even in the face of very real fear of just such a thing happening. Words of assurance about not being rejected by God or isolated from God should be steadily strengthened by the presence of the pastoral caregiver as well as others from the church family.

Secondly, beyond the AIDS patient lies an entire additional area of ministry, which some writers and researchers call the "second epidemic." This epidemic includes all those persons who have not been formally diagnosed with AIDS but who have deep fears that they are carrying the virus in their systems. Many may have been diagnosed as having ARC, or AIDS-Related Complex, where the virus is present but the classic symptoms of full-blown disease have not appeared. There are unsettling expectations of increased incidents of suicide among those caught in this second epidemic.

AIDS experts are projecting large numbers of new cases of this disease in future. It is almost impossible to pick up any national publication or daily newspaper that does not include references to the dilemma of AIDS. The estimate from the Surgeon General alone is that by 1991 we will see some 270,000 cases of AIDS diagnosed.[9] What is more unsettling is the projection that, in our nation today, somewhere around 1.5 million people are already carrying the virus in their systems, though it has yet to become manifest in a way that can be easily diagnosed.[10] That projection, coupled with spreading knowledge about the ways the disease is transmitted, means that there is going to be a huge mass of people out there, many of them sitting in our pews on Sunday, who are living with the fear of coming down with the disease as a result of past sexual activity.

Another consequence of AIDS is becoming evident in some very concrete day-to-day pastoral tasks. For instance, to those couples who have been sexually active and are now choosing marriage and seeking preparation for that relationship, AIDS now brings a whole new dimension.

With the vast amount of sexual freedom we have known in this country since the early sixties, all sorts of fear, anxiety, guilt, and uneasiness are becoming very apparent. The man or woman who had one or more adulterous or promiscuous relationships five or six years ago and is now happily married may wonder each day if he or she contracted AIDS during that time. Or how about the young person who in the confusion of adolescence was involved in some brief homosexual activity before settling into a heterosexual identity and marriage? The panic can become as contagious as AIDS itself. The list could go on and on, but the point is clear. The so-called sexual revolution of recent years is suddenly being seen in a different light in the presence of AIDS.

Some couples do not mind discussing their past sexual experiences. Others feel that the past is best left undisturbed. Either way, the presence of AIDS creates a new dynamic for potential marriages these days. It raises an ethical question as to what needs to be disclosed in terms of what a spouse and the children born in that relationship have a right to know. At this point, there are no clear answers. Since most people are still choosing to be married by a minister in this country, the issue creates both a dilemma and opportunity for premarital counseling.

The sexual implications of AIDS will present new and difficult problems in daily family relationships. Pastors and other staff ministers need to be sensitive to what is going on in their church communities. What may look like job-related stress or marital difficulty or adolescent acting out may instead be rooted in unresolved guilt or anger coming out of a deep fear of contracting or having contracted AIDS. The scope and ramifications of such a dilemma are almost overwhelming. Through sensitive pastoral ministry, the church can become a caring and redemptive community in ways that it has never before explored.

Preaching

One of the very best ways to set the stage for such conversation with the congregation is to address the issue from the pulpit. Some pastors have chosen to devote an entire sermon to the issue of AIDS. This kind of prophetic preaching is difficult and means very thorough preparation on the minister's part. The strength of this approach is that it focuses all the worship energy on a single topic, which is addressed forcefully from a biblical perspective. The weakness of this approach is that it is too easy for the minister or congregation to conclude that, because the subject has been addressed, it has been dealt with and disposed of.

I chose not to devote an entire sermon to the issue of AIDS for two reasons. First of all, we were already dealing with AIDS in the congregation before I became aware that preaching on the subject was important. Given the fact that we were going to be dealing with a support ministry over the long haul, it seemed best to make short references to AIDS in a number of sermons. I used illustrations about AIDS and my own ministry to AIDS patients to underscore and illustrate themes like acceptance of people regardless of who they are, the necessity of taking risks, the transcendence of agape love across all sorts of barriers, and the need for unconditional love to be given. On more than one occasion I raised the issue of the relationship between moral values, especially in the context of sexuality, and the presence of AIDS. I posed to our church the question of what it means when the bulk of discussion these days about safety in sex, as in monogamous relationships, is coming from the medical community in response to a life-threatening disease and not from the church in response to the call of God to live out of an ethical and moral base that is biblical.

The second reason I chose the illustrative approach rather than a single sermon is because of the basic nature and personality of this church. We are not and have never been a "one issue" church. We have tried to respond to whatever came to us in the broader context of ministry, not taking an identity from our response to a single specific issue. It seemed more natural for us to include our response to AIDS as a part of the ongoing process of who we were and are becoming as a church.

Congregational Involvement

The task of responding to AIDS is primarily that of the pastor or minister because this is where the leadership role in the church basically resides. However, no minister can assume responsibility for the response of the entire church. Any minister who enables the congregation to respond jointly will find out what it means to *be* a church community, supporting one another in the common task. Not to do so is to invite personal isolation and pastoral burnout.

Clergy are notorious for claiming more ownership of ministry than is either healthy or even biblical. The many dynamics that are a part of the ministry to AIDS patients and their families almost preclude any minister's being able to mount a Lone Ranger type of response. Ministry in relation to AIDS is a most challenging and difficult task, manageable only when the minister has some support and help in making this journey.

Responding to AIDS in ministry also provides for the

minister an excellent opportunity to live out the concept of ministry as outlined in Ephesians 4:12. In listing the various gifts that were given to those who would function as leaders of the body of Christ, the epistle indicates that all of them focus on one basic task, that of equipping the saints for the work of ministry.

The equipping of the membership of the church for the work of ministry to and with AIDS patients and their families is a normal and biblical outgrowth of the minister's own role. As the minister struggles with his or her response to AIDS, a logical next step is to begin to share with some of the leadership of the church. This could take place informally through normal relationships within the congregation. Nearly all ministers have some sort of informal sounding board in the church community that could be used for this purpose. A more formal approach could be made to the various groups within the church—such as council, deacons, elders, trustees, or missions or outreach committee.

When the minister begins to share his or her concerns with people in the congregation, there is a temptation, with an issue as controversial as AIDS, to be so careful and cautious that the substance of the issue is lost. One is asking permission to deal with the issue rather than claiming ownership of one's own real concern. The minister must always guard against compromising the prophetic role of proclamation. One can honestly express personal concern and, in so doing, invite the congregation to struggle with the issue as well. Once a sense of identity and participation in the issue has been engendered, no permission is needed. What is needed is help and concern from the congregation in responding. Thus, under God's leadership, the congregation can accept, with the minister, the need for ministry to those with AIDS.

Biblical and Moral Context of Involvement

Because it is so closely related to questions of sexual morality, the issue of AIDS is particularly controversial. The

Surgeon General, Dr. C. Everett Koop, has found himself
in the midst of this storm in his steadfast and clear advocacy
of sex education for all and the use of condoms for the
sexually active. He has tried to speak from the perspective
of public health, but his words have been heard in the context of the moral and ethical dimensions of this issue.

For almost two decades, large numbers of people have
followed an open-ended course in terms of sexual practice.
Now the validity of the assumptions underlying this sexual
revolution are being challenged. It is no wonder that Dr.
Koop and others who speak like him are meeting tremendous resistance from many parts of our society.

Many in the church, especially in more conservative
areas, are strongly opposed to the very suggestion of "safer
sex," including the use of condoms, as an appropriate response to the crisis of AIDS. In reality, the religious community will be represented along the entire spectrum of
response to the problem. Some will say that abstinence until
marriage and monogamous sex within marriage is the only
Christian response. Others, more liberal in their ethical and
moral views, will advocate "safer sex" for the sake of public
health. Most of us will be found somewhere between these
two extremes.

The very presence of AIDS within our society means that
the church and its leaders must struggle once again with the
issue of sexuality and sexual practices. In such an effort it
is a real temptation to make the Bible say things more
clearly than perhaps it does, or to confuse what scripture
says with what our society and culture say. Sex is pictured
in various ways in the Bible, each of them reflecting not only
the revelation of God to humankind but also the context of
the time in which specific events happened. Responsible
scholarship would demand that we recognize this and seek
to find the eternal word of truth that speaks to us across
cultures and generations.

For instance, the Song of Songs, infrequently used by
most ministers in preaching, portrays the passionate side of
sex. Some scholars have suggested that this particular book

in the Bible simply glorifies sex in the most human way. The book of Ruth views sex in a totally different way. This little book underscores the naturalness of sex in the context of relationships.

In the Pentateuch, the first five books of the Bible, we find the clearest and perhaps most authoritative word in the Old Testament. Throughout, the major concern regarding sexual relationships is the issue of procreation and childbearing. Recognizing the context—the fragility of the new nation Israel—this is a very understandable position.

In the New Testament, Jesus seems to affirm the Old Testament position of sex being for and in the family. However, the apostle Paul takes a less propitious view in his writings. This is easily understood by his own views about eschatology. Paul lived and ministered in a time when the second coming of Christ was expected on a daily basis. There was a sense of urgency about the end of the world. Therefore, Paul could hardly be completely supportive of the Old Testament view of sex, since it would be unfair to bring children into a world that was going to end in the immediate future. Indeed, it would be inadvisable in Paul's view to enter into any kind of marital or family commitment. It was going to take all of the energy believers had just to prepare for the end of time.

Viewed as a whole, and in the context of the time in which they were written, the scriptures are clear that sex functions best in the context of the marriage relationship. It is in marriage that all parts of the sexual dynamic come together. However, promiscuity and adultery have been and remain a part of the human scene. From the early days of human interaction, our lack of natural monogamy has been apparent. The church has for centuries felt tension in the area of sexuality and sexual practices.

The Christian tradition has maintained that marriage is the place for sex because within marriage the two roles of procreation and union can be fulfilled. Marriage is the best context for creating family, which includes both having and raising children and developing the kind of community as family that reflects the highest kind of biblical relationships.

Until the decade of the eighties, when AIDS appeared in this country, matters of sexuality were mainly topics for theological and moral discussion and deliberation. However clear the church chose to be, the bottom line always rested on the freedom of the individual to choose. It would have been much easier if the church could have dealt with the issue of sex from a rigid biblical or clearly orthodox perspective. However, more often than not, the church found itself on the horns of the dilemma of having to respond to the biblical and moral issues of the freedom of individuals and the fact that their choices and lifestyles may contradict traditional moral values based on the Bible.

Up to now, aside from various venereal diseases, all of which are treatable, the only really destructive threat present in illicit sex was in the area of relationships. (What minister has not dealt with the pain of broken and distorted relationships that have come to the surface because of promiscuous or adulterous sexual activity?) However, the church must recognize that now a new dimension exists because of AIDS; suddenly a whole new light has been thrown on the subject. The issue now is that sex has the potential to kill, not just mess up heads and hearts and relationships.

Promiscuous and adulterous sexuality can kill. That statement alone should enable us to conclude, all other reasons notwithstanding, that promiscuity in today's world is simply stupid. Because the end result of AIDS is death and because of the sheer unknown numbers of humans who unknowingly carry the virus, no intelligent person should be able to pretend that the sexual revolution can continue.

Some will see this as part of the clear judgment and wrath of God on our sexual practices. I continue to struggle with the clear directive, from Jesus himself, that judgment is not my task. That task lies in the area of God's responsibility. Because of that, I don't feel it is appropriate or necessary for me to attempt to identify what is God's judgment and what is not.

Rather, the awareness now that sex can kill people means that I take more seriously than ever the gift from God of freedom of choice in my life. The presence of AIDS puts an entirely new stewardship dimension on the issue of people's freedom. Quite frankly, for the church to focus responsive energy on the simplistic, one-dimensional "say no" response is to miss the point. It is all too easy to seek simple solutions to what is a very complex problem.

The presence of AIDS creates for the church a tremendous opportunity to explore again what are the best and highest kind of relationships that we can have, as we understand the revelation of God. It causes us to look again at our theology of creation as male and female and to discover new insights into what being vulnerable to another human being is all about in this day and age.

In dealing with members of our congregation in Plantation, especially the young people, I have found that the presence of AIDS has created new sensitivity to the old truth that sexuality functions best in the context of the marriage relationship. Sexuality functions best when people take each other seriously in terms of their vulnerability. Sexuality functions best when people do not use one another for their own ends and pleasures. Affirming the traditional position of the church in the area of sexuality is perhaps easier now than it has been in years.

However and wherever the church decides to come down on this particular dimension of the issue theologically and morally, numbers of people will still choose to be sexually active. How will the church in general and its ministers in particular respond to these people? Some will play holy ostrich and simply refuse to see this as a fact of life. Their response will continue to be one-dimensional: abstinence outside of marriage; monogamy inside of marriage. There is another possibility, most dramatically symbolized in the condom. In spite of the best and clearest communication we can offer, there are still some who will say that regardless of the presence of AIDS, wide sexual activity is important to them. Because of this, ministers have a theological obligation to counsel them with whatever means of caution and safety are available.

Once what I believe is the best and highest context for human sexuality has been presented and heard, then biblically I must respect a person's right to choose not to respond in that way. Indeed, if I expect him or her to listen to my position, freely chosen from all the choices I have, then, it seems, I must be willing to respect his or her position. In this context, I would have no difficulty advising the use of condoms in sexual activity as an expression of concern for that person's health and well-being. The issue of public health that the Surgeon General repeatedly emphasizes simply cannot be avoided just because it does not fit into our traditional theological package.

A relevant and contemporary parallel to this response is seen in the development of groups of students in local high schools who are concerned about drunk driving. A very popular organization is known as SADD (Students Against Drunken Driving). Given the reality of alcohol in our society, we have little difficulty understanding SADD's position that indiscriminate and abusive drinking habits linked with driving have the potential to kill. A part of the work of this organization is to get a commitment from the young people themselves, not to drive when drinking and not to let their friends drive when they have been drinking. Parental involvement is also a part of this approach. Parents sign their part of the agreement, stating that if their child drinks inappropriately, the child can call them and the parents will come and take their son or daughter home safely, with no reprisals.

A few people may feel that participation in SADD is a giving of permission to use alcohol in any way or form one wants. It is not. It is a way of recognizing the danger and the reality and respecting the right of individuals to make decisions that we may not agree with or even like. And it reflects the belief that their worth as living individuals is more significant than any other issue.

Likewise, there are those who will see suggesting the use

of condoms as giving permission for sexual activity of any variety. Without a clear word from the church on our best understanding of sexuality from a biblical perspective, perhaps it is. However, when we have sought to use all that God has given us to understand and arrive at a position in a very complex issue, then to suggest the use of condoms as a preventive measure in regard to AIDS seems to be a logical biblical extension of concern for human life.

This whole issue of sexuality and the presence of AIDS cannot be simply dismissed or lightly treated. We must respond to it with preparation, care, and concern. We must be willing to take our positions as clearly as we know how under God's leadership. We must be willing to be available to minister to all who are involved who come our way, whether we agree with them or not. As illogical as it seems, our final place in this dilemma is out by the gate, like the father in Luke's story of the Prodigal, waiting for those who are able to come back from the far country.

Education

The normal organizational life of almost any church abounds with opportunities for an educational effort about AIDS. The focus should be twofold.

Sharing copies of the *Surgeon General's Report on Acquired Immune Deficiency Syndrome* is a strong starting place. Other pamphlets can be obtained from the local American Red Cross office or public health services.

It could be a very healthy and exciting experience to create some role-playing episodes and let the leadership of the church struggle with what the response of the church ought to be. These scenarios could take the form of the various circumstances in which the disease is experienced in our society. Such role plays should be balanced in terms of the context of the disease. One could focus on an AIDS patient who is homosexual, another on an I.V. drug user, another on someone who has contracted the disease through blood transfusions, another on a newborn baby and its mother. Additional scenarios could be about family members—parents whose children have AIDS or spouses or children of AIDS patients. Role-playing can be done in youth or adult groups or in intergenerational groups.

In our church we were fortunate that the relationship between Tom and the young people enabled us to ask him to come to discuss the issue with them as it related to drug use. It was a very draining and brave thing for Tom to want to do, and it most certainly had its impact. To have known him and seen him around the church before he contracted AIDS, and then to listen to him in his weakened condition as he talked about the dangers of drug use and AIDS, was very powerful.

Some churches have taken a more elaborate approach to education about AIDS. An Episcopal congregation in Plantation chose to focus on this issue through its church school for a period of three weeks. The first week, they invited a specialist in infectious diseases to address the medical aspects of the issue. The second week they had a minister come to address the theological and religious concerns, and in the third week they invited a psychiatrist to speak to the emotional and psychological concerns. The series was undertaken to prepare the church for its own response to the presence of AIDS in their community of faith.

Such approaches in preparation could provide some very exciting dialogue and discussion, in that people would be having to struggle with an issue from real life against the background of the meaning and directive in scripture regarding the ministry to persons in need. Any church that responds to AIDS should be resolutely assured of their firm biblical basis for action. For a minister and people to struggle authentically with real-life issues in the context of biblical rationale for response is a most stimulating growth experience. One of the bottom-line questions in this process is, "Will the gospel work in the face of something like AIDS?" Another way to phrase that is, "Will the church be the church when AIDS comes on the scene?"

It would be most helpful to have these kinds of discussions and experiences *before* AIDS comes to church. To be proactive is always a stronger way to go than being reactive. Our own congregation had to spend the bulk of its energy playing catch-up to what was already happening. There are places where we could have been greatly strengthened by having discussed some of this together before the fact.

To deal with the issue before the fact also means that the discussion is free of the complications of confidentiality. This in itself will make struggling with the subject of AIDS much more manageable. Discussions and responses can be totally open and have no risk of being colored by the presence of AIDS already in the congregation.

If, however, AIDS in the congregation is what gives rise to discussions between minister and congregation, there can be the same kind of exploration of possibilities. It will just have to take place with a bit of caution in regard to confidentiality. In addition, it is important to be sure that one particular incidence of AIDS does not become the focal point of concern for response. Because of the probability that AIDS will reoccur, care needs to be exercised to assure consideration of the broadest kinds of possibilities.

For instance, if the first case of AIDS that appeared in a church congregation was due to drug-related activity, it is important to remember that other kinds of causes are possible. There could be cases of AIDS arising out of homosexual or bisexual relationships. There could also be cases resulting from adultery or promiscuity. I cannot overemphasize how important it is not to draw conclusions about ministering to persons with AIDS on the basis of the context in which the disease was contracted.

Congregational Policies

Out of these discussions, which are in themselves an ongoing educational process, could come the clarification of positions and policies for the church. For instance, what will be the reaction of the church with regard to the nursery should AIDS come to church? The question of letting children with AIDS remain in schools and churches has become a highly emotional issue in many communities. It would seem a wise use of time and energy to gather the children's workers or nursery workers together with a medical resource person—perhaps a nurse or a doctor—who could talk candidly about the risks to other children. While most people are sympathetic to young victims of this disease, such as hemophiliacs, a high level of uneasiness still arises about the possibility of their children being in the same room with a child with AIDS. Issues such as the sharing of toys that little children inevitably put in their mouths in the nursery, or the possibility that a child with AIDS might cut and bleed onto another child with a small open sore or scratch, are very real in the minds of parents. Time spent in the development of a plan of action for such circumstances would be most helpful if it were done before an actual situation arose, so that the personalities of the sick children and their families would not be involved.

Even though the medical community has consistently and repeatedly said that AIDS is not transmitted casually in such settings, fears nonetheless persist. Even though most school systems that have faced this issue have decided to keep AIDS-related children in the mainstream of classes, parents still fear for their own children. The issue has the potential of creating real division within a church community. Therefore, it is very important to discuss and prepare for it before the fact, if at all possible.

The same issue may arise in the Sunday school or in other organizational activities that in any way might touch the lives of those who are dealing with AIDS. The church, in responding in ministry to those with AIDS and their families, should not need to form sudden policies or positions as a reaction to crisis. Careful thought should be given to these issues for the larger context of the church community, and any policy or position established must come from an authentic biblical context.

In addition to the biblical teaching discussed earlier, several other basic elements need to be considered in policy dicussions, in the context of relationships in the congregation and community.

1. The church needs to recognize that any new policy should be a natural outgrowth of a thorough study of the whole issue of AIDS. To fail to do so is to risk formulation of a policy based on collective ignorance or hearsay rather than on facts.

2. Any policy that is adopted is at the same time a bold public statement about the theology of a given congregation—a faith statement of the church's understanding of the nature of God, the relationship of God to people, and the theological basis of relationship between persons.

3. Any congregation considering an AIDS policy needs to be very sure that the policy addresses the real underlying issue of sexual behavior. While most policies *seem* to address the issue of contagion and *seem* to be designed to protect the healthy members of the congregation, many of them spring from a deep-seated discomfort with sexual matters. Since a large number of documented AIDS cases are related to sexual transmission, the sexual factor is very apt to be the driving force in policy formation.

4. Any policy concerning AIDS needs to take into account the continuing development of legal opinion and precedent. To date, most of the litigation in the religious community has been around the area of confidentiality. Questions are yet to be considered regarding the relationship of rights and responsibilities of membership in a congregation to a special new policy about AIDS.

5. Any policy regarding AIDS must be consistent with other policies. For instance, if policies about AIDS arise because for theological reasons a congregation does not want to include persons who represent what they have determined to be "sinful" behavior, what about policies for other kinds of behavior that could be defined biblically as sinful? If policies arise because of fear of contagion, what about policies for other infectious diseases? If policies are developed because of the life-threatening nature of AIDS,

what about policies regarding other terminal diseases? Consistency is a most important issue.

After three years of living with AIDS in our congregation, First Baptist Church of Plantation decided that no special policy is necessary. Even in our children's and nursery areas, we feel that our present policies on illness and hygiene are sufficient. Should we be faced with additional circumstances in the future, we can give further consideration to the matter.

Support Groups

One of the most needed kinds of ministry is providing a welcoming place in which persons with AIDS can find a support group during their illness. The church might even provide skilled leadership in the area of psychology or counseling for such groups from within its own membership. While just providing space may be the most needed thing, there will also be other more specific needs to which groups within the church can respond.

The ministry of South Main Baptist Church in Houston, Texas, embodies several of these aspects. As an outgrowth of an ongoing social ministry of the church, support groups were begun for AIDS patients, led by one of their members who works as a counselor in a local psychiatric hospital. In addition, they are trying to respond to the needs of families of persons with AIDS. They have found that it is more difficult to reach some families than it is to minister to the patients themselves. Many families are uneasy about being identified with AIDS. Again, the issue of confidentiality is very significant. One of the ways South Main has found to minister to families is to be able to provide housing for them when they come to Houston to visit with family members who are hospitalized. Many in the church open their own homes to these visiting family members during this time. The response of this church has also taken the form of meeting very real physical needs of persons with AIDS. As a part of their already existing food pantry and feeding program, members have worked together to prepare and deliver food to AIDS patients. Regular ongoing visitation to persons with AIDS, both at home and in the hospital, is also a part of their ministry.

When needs are really individual, as in special diets that the food pantry cannot supply, funds from the church make possible the purchase of what is needed for a given patient. The name of this overall ministry at South Main is FOCUS, short for Focus On Caring, Understanding, and Support. In an interview, the pastor of that church summed it up: "We're here to minister to patients and their families. Our FOCUS ministry realizes that the larger moral imperative is to minister 'to the least of these' as Jesus commanded."[11]

Special attention must be given to the need for support groups for family members. These could be organized for the whole family, including spouses, children, and parents of AIDS patients. Other times, consideration would need to be given to groups for specific family members. The size of the population affected by AIDS will determine the configuration of these groups. If the numbers in a given geographical area were sufficient, there could be real value in a group just for the children of AIDS patients, or just for spouses or parents. (Remember the description in chapter 4 of how a support group was formed for Ruth.)

Hospice Care

There are any number of possibilities, especially in larger congregations, for the structuring of responses to meet some of the most significant needs that AIDS patients have. This is particularly true for those who have no families to care for them and no resources to obtain care for themselves. Many AIDS patients are in this category, having lost their jobs and accompanying insurance benefits. Much of the ongoing illness associated with AIDS is such that constant hospitalization is not required, but living alone is also not an option.

One church in our community gathered several members

and formed a nonprofit corporation in order to secure some apartments that could be made available to AIDS patients. The group also provides assistance in living skills as well as making sure that medical contacts are available, along with ongoing counseling. This approach would certainly be possible if several churches were to work together by pooling both leadership and financial resources. Nearly every expert in the field of AIDS tells us that the present medical system will simply not be able to handle the financial load of patient care, to say nothing of other needs. Sources within the nonprofit sector of society have a wonderful opportunity to meet a real need. The church, in particular, has the opportunity to apply to dealing with AIDS its know-how gained in such fields as service to older people and children. While this response to AIDS is a bit more extensive and complicated, it nonetheless must be seen as a viable and important alternative to consider.

Special Projects

In those areas where there are centers that focus on ministry to persons with AIDS, it is relatively easy to discover ways that groups from a church can be involved. Where there is no AIDS center as such, you might check with a hospice program, which more than likely will have AIDS patients under its care. You might also contact a chaplain at one of the larger hospitals in your area that would deal with AIDS patients. Any such source should be able to suggest ways to be involved in some kind of ministry. As a result of such contacts, several of our members in Plantation quietly go about the task of regular hospital visitations to AIDS patients.

Another timely way to focus the life of a congregation on the issue of AIDS is to designate a given day as a day of prayer for all those who are suffering with the disease. Prayers for families of AIDS patients need to be clearly focused as well. This is a relatively simple yet profound way to raise the consciousness of a congregation. At the same time, groundwork is laid for whatever might evolve later in terms of ministry or response. Some churches have even ended this kind of day with a brief candlelight service. Such a service could be built around the theme of the power and value of intercessory prayer. It would even be appropriate to provide an opportunity to identify specific concerns of members of the congregation regarding individuals they know who have AIDS.

One of the most significant and interesting events in our congregation took place just before Christmas of 1986. Our church always tries to focus on some sort of special ministry around Christmas, such as food or toys for those for whom such things would be a special gift. The director of the local AIDS center indicated that they always had a need for bed sheets. The center operates a small unit for AIDS patients who have nowhere else to go during their illness. The presence of high fevers and night sweats means frequent changes of bed linen. Our church chose to take on the project for our Christmas emphasis.

We decided that ample publicity was needed and we would designate a given Sunday as AIDS Sheet Sunday. We chose the Sunday just before Christmas, feeling that the numbers of people in attendance would be high. We requested each family coming to church that day to bring a set of single sheets and a pillowcase and deposit them in a large box we placed in the vestibule of our sanctuary. It was important, symbolically, that the giving of sheets take place in the sanctuary as a part of coming to worship, so people would connect giving with what worship is all about. We were not only pleased with the number of sheets we received but also with the serious way our folks responded. Many of them were planning to be out of town for Christmas, and it was a moving experience to see the number of additional sheets that were brought personally to the church office the week before Christmas. Others who were not going to be there simply brought in checks, with which we purchased sheets in bulk to be added to those already brought in. The special offering was a powerful and significant way to relate a real need about a vital issue like AIDS to an entire congregation at a very special time of the year.

Caring for the Caregiver

By the very nature of the disease, a response to AIDS can be an all-consuming thing. It is very easy to get so caught up in the scope of this disease, in the pain it causes, both physical and emotional, and in its demands, that one fails to keep a sense of balance. Anyone who begins to respond to AIDS in ministry needs to remember the importance of normalcy. Daily, often repetitive, ever-present tasks have been some of the best gifts I have had. Ministering to AIDS patients and their families is exhausting. On more than one occasion, the last thing I wanted to do afterward was go home and wash the dog, cut the grass, prepare a sermon, write an article for the church newsletter, or anything else— everything seemed to pale into insignificance in light of the tragedy of AIDS. However, it is these normal tasks that enable us, not only to keep our sanity but to keep a sense of balance in what we are about. They serve to remind us that, in the economy of God, all things have an importance. For me to get so caught up in one issue or ministry to the exclusion of other things is for me to deem unimportant what God has deemed important. I am learning to look with a sense of eagerness to those things in my life and ministry that lend normalcy and balance. They in no way detract from what I am called upon to do in response to AIDS. In fact, they enhance my effectiveness as a whole person who is struggling with a response of ministry to those with AIDS and their families.

Pastors like to pretend that their source of energy and resources is limitless. They believe that, because they are God's servants, God will provide for their every need. But God also allows us to find out for ourselves that we, too, are human. We get tired and depressed; we become confused and even angry. There is always the chance of making some really bad judgment calls because of fatigue and weariness. As ministers we are often guilty of not being good stewards of the energy and health that God has given us.

Dealing with AIDS patients and their families over an extended period of time can be particularly draining, as I learned after walking with several families through the valley of death from AIDS. Subtle depression creeps up, and before you know it you can find yourself overwhelmed.

In ministering with Tom and Ruth, I invested a tremendous amount of personal energy in their journey. Not only was Tom a close friend, the pressure of pulling this book together heightened my involvement. As the time for his death neared, I began to realize that I was almost in over my head in terms of my own emotional resources. There was the realization that after all we had been through, he was going to die anyway. The subsequent need to conduct a funeral and be a strong spiritual leader was almost more than I could handle. Where could I go with my own pain? Who was going to care for the caregiver?

In the midst of my grief, I did two things that turned out to be very redemptive. First, I talked with a friend who is a counselor. He provided me with some clearer vision of my abilities and my limitations. Second, I turned to the men and women of our deacon council and requested their prayers and concern for me as we walked through the death experience with Tom and Ruth. I also shared this concern with the church family as a whole in our midweek prayer service.

Many ministers might feel that such a move is a mistake. To share one's weaknesses or fears would seem to undercut one's ability to function as a spiritual leader. I found quite the opposite to be true. In fact, if anything, my leadership was enhanced by honestly sharing my needs as well as acknowledging the needs of others.

However you choose to do it is up to you. Do it privately or in small groups or with your entire congregation. But do not pretend that you will not have your own needs to be cared for during these journeys. It is crucial for you to be mature enough to let those in the body of Christ around you provide care for you, the caregiver.

All of us, whether minister or lay person, can identify with the feelings of uneasiness and fear about participating in an area of life that seems so new and unknown. We all need to be reminded that fears in relation to ministry have always been a part of the saga of humankind. The Genesis account of creation depicts movement away from the ideal that God had set before man and woman. After eating the forbidden fruit, Adam and Eve hid themselves when God came looking for them, because they were afraid (Genesis 3). From the New Testament perspective, the good news is that, in the midst of such heavy reality, God himself has come to pitch his tent among us (John 1) and journey with us, showing us the way and shouldering the burden with us as we go.

For those with AIDS and their families, the Word of God indeed becomes flesh again and again as the church reaches out and ministers to those in need. There is no situation in which people are more desperate to hear "good news" than that concerning AIDS. I pray that our need to judge will be laid aside as we discover our need to minister, regardless of lifestyle or circumstance. I pray that our human inclination to avoid risky or difficult tasks will be transformed into the courage to be present in the strong name of Jesus Christ, wherever there is need. I pray that those who are walking each day through the dark, dark valley of AIDS will find a sense of direction and a peace that does indeed pass understanding, because the church is willing to be the church.

Epilogue

The journey continues. After three years of ministry to the families within our congregation who are dealing with AIDS, I find myself wishing that this could be the last chapter of the story of this disease, for those who have suffered and lost, for the church which has struggled, and for me as a pastor. Unfortunately, such will not be the case. If the projections are correct, we have only begun to see what is ahead for all of us. It will be a difficult and a complicated journey. It is one, I fear, that will become an inevitable part of the pastoral landscape of the future.

The journey itself is very demanding. The fact that it always ends in death makes it even more burdensome. I hope and pray that this part of the picture will change and some medical treatment will be found. Until that time, we must just keep on.

Of the four families in our church who have been touched by the disease, all but one have been to the cemetery and are now trying to get life back together again. Late in 1984, Dennis introduced me to AIDS through the death of his grandson. Tom and Ruth were next, with Tom's diagnosis in early 1985. Our journey with him was the most intense, in that he was the only church member who had AIDS. The other situations involved members of the church who had someone in their family with the disease.

Tom's response to AIDS was a singular testimony to his faith and to being a participant in honest ministry. Tom lived almost two and a half years with the disease after diagnosis, longer than the average, which is about eighteen months. (Most patients with AIDS deal with two or three rounds of *Pneumocystis carinii* pneumonia before dying. Tom went through five bouts before dying on June 2, 1987.) On more than one occasion, Tom told me that being part of a church community that chose to accept him as he was, AIDS and all, was life-giving in a literal sense. We miss him terribly. Our lives and our church will never be the same after having known this man and his journey. Part of his calmness and readiness for death came from the security he felt in knowing that Ruth would continue to be a part of this community of faith. The bonds formed during those long months of illness will continue throughout her lifetime.

Ruth expressed her appreciation in a statement made at the close of worship on October 18, 1987. She concluded her comments by saying, "You have showed that you are not afraid to deal with whatever issue comes along and deal with it all the way, the same way Jesus would have. And today I come to celebrate a new birth and I want all of you to join in my celebration. After finding myself immobilized and unable to go on with my life or even to finish mourning, I finally found the strength and courage to be tested for the HIV virus. Much to my surprise and I think to many others as well, my test results were negative. With this new lease on life, I come here today to tell you all how much I love you and to thank you all for loving me."

Larry had family in our church who took seriously the loneliness and isolation he was facing in the spiritual dimension of his journey. Although Larry entered our ministry here at First Baptist Church after Tom and Ruth, he died first, on December 27, 1986, just two days after Christmas.

Elaine and her family are the last to date to be a part of this story. Her husband has AIDS. Though still married, they are separated, and Elaine spends every available moment seeking to be helpful to him. She is awaiting what the others have already gone through. While she waits, she deals with her frustration, anger, and pain at the way this disease literally sucks the life out of those it infects. As her pastor and her church, we wait with her through these dark days that precede the coming death of her husband.

At this point there are no operations, no medications, and no treatments that can offer hope that there is a way to have AIDS and not die. Until that time comes, we must take the best of what science and medicine give us and join it with those transcendent gifts of the church, acceptance, love, faithfulness, and hope. We must continue to commit ourselves to persistent and sensitive ministry to all who need us, patients or family members, regardless of their identity or their past experiences. Faithful or unfaithful, gay or straight, druggie or clean, promiscuous or monogamous, all need to hear the compassionate good news of the love of God, fully revealed in Jesus Christ and manifest in his body, the church.

A final word comes from my experience on the day Tom died. Ruth had called early that morning to say she felt the end was near and she and Tom wanted me to be there with them. Driving over to their home, I looked over to the west, and there was the most magnificent rainbow that I had seen in a long time. It was complete, horizon to horizon and filled the sky with its brightness. I thought to myself, as I neared Tom's house, how ironic it was, to be going to be with someone who was dying of AIDS and, as I went, to find in the sky the serendipitous surprise of a rainbow. Suddenly the irony changed to a feeling of perfect harmony as I recalled the story of the first rainbow God placed in the sky after the great flood, survived only by Noah and his family and animals on the ark.

I felt the rainbow reaffirmed that God was finished with trying to deal with humankind through destruction and fear and punishment and judgment. God once more had hung these magnificent colors across the morning sky. As I pulled into the driveway and prepared to go into the house to wait as my dear friend and brother died, I went with the bold assurance that our journey together had been good. It had been the way of God in struggling with acceptance and love and justice. It had indeed been the way of the rainbow.

Appendix

AIDS Hotline Numbers (Toll free)

U.S. Public Health Service AIDS Hotline   1-800-342-2437

National Sexually Transmitted Diseases
Hotline/American Social Health Association 1-800-227-8922

National Gay Task Force AIDS Information   1-800-221-7044
  Hotlines   1-212-529-1604

AIDS Information from State Departments of Health

Alabama: 205-261-5131
Alaska: 907-561-4406
Arizona: 602-255-1203
Arkansas: 501-661-2395
California: 916-445-0553
Colorado: 303-331-8320
Connecticut: 203-549-6789
Delaware: 302-995-8422
District of Columbia:
  202-332-AIDS
Florida: 904-488-2905
Georgia: 800-342-2437
Hawaii: 808-735-5303
Idaho: 208-334-5944
Illinois: 312-871-5696
Indiana: 317-633-8406
Iowa: 515-281-5424

Kansas: 913-862-9360
Kentucky: 502-564-4478
Louisiana: 504-342-6711
Maine: 207-289-3747
Maryland: 301-945-AIDS
Massachusetts: 617-727-0368
Michigan: 517-335-8371
Minnesota: 612-623-5414
Mississippi: 601-354-6660
Missouri: 816-353-9902
Montana: 406-444-4740
Nebraska: 402-471-2937
Nevada: 702-885-4988 or
  5948
New Hampshire:
  603-271-4487
New Jersey: 609-588-3520

New Mexico: 505-984-0911
New York: 518-473-0641
North Carolina:
  919-733-3419
North Dakota: 701-224-2378
Ohio: 614-466-4643
Oklahoma: 405-271-4061
Oregon: 503-229-5792
Pennsylvania: 717-787-3350
Rhode Island: 401-277-2362
South Carolina: 803-734-5482

South Dakota: 605-773-3364
Tennessee: 615-741-7247
Texas: 512-458-7504
Utah: 801-538-6191
Vermont: 802-863-7240
Virginia: 804-786-6267
Washington: 206-361-2914
West Virginia: 304-348-5358
Wisconsin: 608-267-3583
Wyoming: 307-777-7953

Additional AIDS Information

National

U.S. Public Health Service Public Affairs Office   1-202-245-6867
Hubert H. Humphrey Building, Room 725-H
200 Independence Avenue SW
Washington, DC 20201

American Red Cross   1-202-737-8300
AIDS Education Office
1730 D Street NW
Washington, DC 20006

American Association of Physicians
  for Human Rights   1-415-558-9353
P.O. Box 14366
San Francisco, CA 94114

AIDS Action Council   1-202-547-3101
729 Eighth Street SE, Suite 200
Washington, DC 20003

Centers for Disease Control   1-800-342-2437
U.S. Public Health Service

Gay Men's Health Crisis   1-212-807-6655
P.O. Box 274
132 West 24th Street
New York, NY 10011

Hispanic AIDS Forum   1-212-870-1902
c/o APRED   1-212-870-1864
853 Broadway, Suite 2007
New York, NY 10003

Lambda Legal Defense and Education Fund   1-212-944-9488
132 West 43rd Street, 5th Floor
New York, NY 10036

Los Angeles AIDS Project   1-213-871-2437
1362 Santa Monica Boulevard
Los Angeles, CA 90046

Minority Task Force on AIDS   1-212-749-1214
c/o New York City Council of Churches
475 Riverside Drive, Room 456
New York, NY 10115

Mothers of AIDS Patients (MAP)   1-619-234-3432
c/o Barbara Peabody
3403 E Street
San Diego, CA 92102

National AIDS Network   1-202-546-2424
729 Eighth Street, SE, Suite 300
Washington, DC 20003

National Association of People with AIDS   1-202-483-7979
P.O. Box 65472
Washington, DC 20035

National Coalition of Gay Sexually
   Transmitted Diseases Services   1-414-277-7671
c/o Mark Behar
P.O. Box 239
Milwaukee, WI 53201

National Council of Churches/AIDS
   Task Force   1-212-870-2421
475 Riverside Drive, Room 572
New York, NY 10115

National Hemophilia Foundation   1-212-219-8180
Soho Building
110 Green Street, Room 406
New York, NY 10012

National Institute of Allergy and Infectious
    Diseases   1-301-496-5717
Office of Research Reporting and Public Response

National Lesbian and Gay Health Foundation   1-202-797-3708
P.O. Box 65472
Washington, DC 20035

San Francisco AIDS Foundation   1-415-863-2437
333 Valencia Street, 4th Floor
San Francisco, CA 94103

Local

California
California Department of Health Services   1-916-445-0553
AIDS Activities
P.O. Box 160146
Sacramento, CA 95816-0146

AIDS Project/Los Angeles   1-213-871-1284
837 North Cole Street, Suite 3
Los Angeles, CA 90038

San Diego AIDS Project   1-619-294-2437
4304 Third Avenue
P.O. Box 81082
San Diego, CA 92138

San Francisco AIDS Foundation   1-415-864-4376
333 Valencia Street, 4th Floor
San Francisco, CA 94103

Colorado
Colorado AIDS Project   1-303-837-0166
P.O. Box 18529
Denver, CO 80218

District of Columbia
AIDS Action Project   1-202-332-5295
Whitman-Walker Clinic   1-202-332-2437
2335 18th Street NW
Washington, DC 20009

St. Francis Center   1-202-234-5613
3800 Macomb Street NW
Washington, DC 20016

Florida
AIDS Center One   1-305-561-0316
370 East Prospect
Ft. Lauderdale, FL 33334

AIDS Education Project   1-305-294-8302
P.O. Box 4073
Key West, FL 33041

Health Crisis Network   1-305-634-4636
P.O. Box 52-1546
Miami, FL 33152

Georgia
AID Atlanta (AIDA)   1-404-872-0600
1132 West Peachtree Street NW, Suite 112
Atlanta, GA 30309

Hawaii
Life Foundation   1-808-537-2211
320 Ward Avenue, Suite 104
Honolulu, HI 96814

Illinois
Howard Brown Memorial Clinic   1-312-871-5777
2676 N. Halsted Street
Chicago, IL 60614

Louisiana
Foundation for Health Education   1-504-244-6900
P.O. Box 51537
New Orleans, LA 70151

Maryland
Health Education Resource Center   1-301-945-2437
101 West Read Street, Suite 819
Baltimore, MD 21201

Massachusetts
Fenway Community Health Center   1-617-267-7573
AIDS Action Committee
16 Haviland Street
Boston, MA 02215

Michigan
United Community Services   1-313-833-0622
51 West Warren Avenue
Detroit, MI 48201

Minnesota
Minnesota AIDS Project   1-612-824-1772
P.O. Box 300122
Minneapolis, MN 55403

New York
New York City Health Department (Hot Line)   1-718-485-8111

Gay Men's Health Crisis   1-212-807-6655
P.O. Box 274
132 West 24th Street
New York, NY 10011

Ohio
Health Issues Task Force   1-216-651-1448
P.O. Box 14925, Public Square Station
Cleveland, OH 44114

Oregon
Cascade AIDS Project   1-503-223-8299
408 SW Second Avenue, Suite 403
Portland, OR 97204

Pennsylvania
Philadelphia Community Health Alternatives   1-215-624-2879
Philadelphia AIDS Task Force
P.O. Box 7259
Philadelphia, PA 19109

Tennessee
Lifestyle Health Services   1-615-329-1478
1729 Church Street
Nashville, TN 37203 .

Texas
KS/AIDS Foundation   .   1-713-524-2437
3317 Montrose, Box 1155
Houston, TX 77006

Virginia
Richmond AIDS Information Network   1-804-358-6343
Fan Free Clinic
1721 Hanover Avenue
Richmond, VA 23220

Washington
Northwest AIDS Foundation   1-206-326-4166
P.O. Box 3449
Seattle, WA 98114

Wisconsin
Brady East STD Clinic   1-414-273-2437
Milwaukee AIDS Project
1240 East Brady Street
Milwaukee, WI 53202

Canada
AIDS Committee Toronto (ACT)   1-416-926-1626
P.O. Box 55, Station F
Toronto M4Y 2L4, Ontario
Canada

Notes

1. *Surgeon General's Report on Acquired Immune Deficiency Syndrome* (Washington, D.C.: U.S. Government Printing Office, 1986), p. 12.
2. Ibid.
3. *Surgeon General's Report,* p. 6.
4. Ibid., *Surgeon General's Report,* p. 15.
5. Fort Lauderdale *Sun Sentinel,* March 4, 1987.
6. *Surgeon General's Report,* p. 5.
7. Frederick Buechner, *Wishful Thinking* (New York: Harper & Row, 1973), p. 48.
8. Victor Gong and Norman Rudnick, eds., *AIDS: Facts and Issues* (New Brunswick, N.J.: Rutgers University Press, 1986), p. 278.
9. *Surgeon General's Report,* p. 6.
10. Ibid., p. 12.
11. *Baptist Press,* November 11, 1986.